Healthy
BEGINNINGS

4th edition

{ Giving your baby the best start,
from **preconception to birth**. }

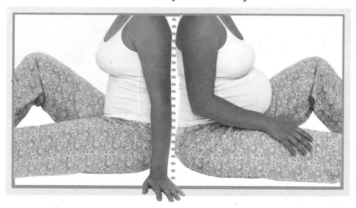

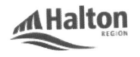

Baby & Parent
Health

KEY QUESTIONS TO ASK WHEN A TEST, TREATMENT OR INTERVENTION IS SUGGESTED
Adapted from Penny Simkin

1. What is the reason for this? Why is it needed?
2. How is it done? How likely is it to be useful/successful?
3. Are there any further steps after this?
4. Are there any risks or side effects?
5. Are there any alternatives? (including waiting or doing nothing) If yes, ask the above questions regarding the alternative(s).

In an emergency, it may be impossible to fully explore these questions. Your caregiver should tell you how serious and urgent the situation is.

Healthy
BEGINNINGS

4th edition

Giving your baby the best start,
from **preconception to birth**.

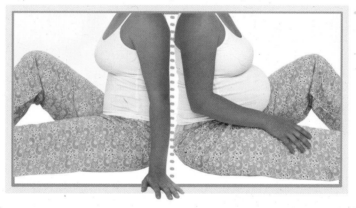

Nan Schuurmans, MD, FRCSC, Edmonton, AB under the direction of
Vyta Senikas, MDCM, FRCSC, Associate Executive Vice-President, SOGC, Ottawa, ON
and André B. Lalonde, MD, FRCSC, Executive Vice-President, SOGC, Ottawa, ON

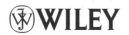

WILEY

John Wiley & Sons Canada, Ltd.

Production Credits

Edited by:	Stuart Adams
Designed by:	Red Wagon Studio
Illustrations:	Julie Dorion
Copy editor:	Susan James
Cover:	Red Wagon Studio
Cover Photos:	Creative Concepts Photography
Typesetting:	Thomson Digital
Printer:	Printcrafters

Library and Archives Canada Cataloguing in Publication

Schuurmans, Nan

    Healthy beginnings : giving your baby the best start, from preconception to birth / [written by Nan Schuurmans ; under the direction of Vyta Senikas and André Lalonde ; illustrations, Julie Dorion]. — 4th ed.

Includes index.
ISBN 978-0-470-16024-4
ISBN 978-0-470-73626-5

1. Pregnancy—Miscellanea. 2. Childbirth—Miscellanea. 3. Infants
    (Newborn)—Care—Miscellanea. I. Lalonde, André, 1943- II. Society of
    Obstetricians and Gynaecologists of Canada III. Title.

RG525.S34 2006   618.2   C2005-907545-7

John Wiley & Sons Canada, Ltd.
6045 Freemont Blvd.
Mississauga, Ontario
L5R 4J3

This book is printed with biodegradable vegetable-based inks on 60lb. recycled white paper, 100% post-consumer waste.

© **Mixed Sources**
Product group from well-managed forests, controlled sources and recycled wood or fiber
www.fsc.org Cert no. SW-COC-002520
FSC © 1996 Forest Stewardship Council

Printed in Canada

2 3 4 5 PC 13 12 11 10

This book reflects current knowledge and evidence-based practice. The information should not be construed as dictating an exclusive course of treatment or procedure to be followed. Your health-care provider should be consulted and will advise you on your pregnancy and (or) specific problems. The authors, publishers, printer, and others contributing to the preparation of this document cannot accept liability for errors, omissions, or any consequences arising from the use of the information.

Table of contents

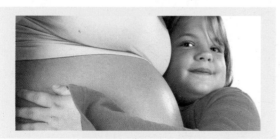

CHAPTER THREE
Gentle growth: the second trimester

CHAPTER FOUR
The home stretch: the third trimester

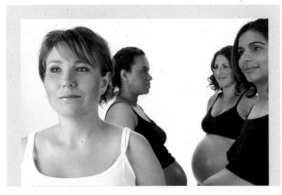

Acknowledgements

Healthy Beginnings: Giving your baby the best start, from preconception to birth. 4th edition. Based on the SOGC's clinical practice guidelines.

The Society of Obstetricians and Gynaecologists of Canada would like to thank the following organizations for their help:

Best Start: Ontario's Maternal, Newborn, and Early Child Development Resource Centre by Health Nexus

Canadian Paediatric Society

CAMH – PREGNETs

Central South West Reproductive Health Working Group

Centre for Addiction and Mental Health

Diabetes Ontario

Halton Region Health Department

Health Canada: Hélène Lowell, RD, Office of Nutrition Policy and Promotion

Infant Mental Health Promotion

Montreal Diet Dispensary Dietitians: Marie-Paule Duquette, Émilie Masson, and Karen Medeiros

Motherisk

Ontario Breastfeeding Committee

Ottawa Public Health

Peterborough County-City Health Unit

Plain language editing of this book was done by Debra Isabel Huron, under auspices of the Plain Language Service at the Canadian Public Health Association

Registered Nurses Association of Ontario

Women's College Hospital, Sport C.A.R.E.

The Society of Obstetricians and Gynaecologists of Canada would like to thank the following individuals for their help:

Julia M.K. Alleyne, BHsc(PT), MD, CCFP, Dip. Sport Med., Toronto, ON
Jon Barrett, MD, FRCOG, FRCSC, Toronto, ON
Irene Colliton, MD, Edmonton, AB
Martina Delaney, MD, St. John's, NL
Lillian Dunn, RM, Thunder Bay, ON
Brenda Dushinski, RN, Calgary, AB
Ahmed Ezzat, MD, FRCSC, Saskatoon, SK
Mark Feldman, MD, FRCPC, Toronto, ON
Guy-Paul Gagné, MD, FRCSC, LaSalle, QC
Michael Helewa, MD, FRCSC, Winnipeg, MB
Nancy Huggett, Ottawa, ON
Gideon Koren, MD, FRCPC, FACMT, Toronto, ON
Dean Leduc, MD, Ottawa, ON
Laura A. Magee, MD, Vancouver, BC
Deborah Money, MD, FRCSC, Vancouver, BC
Patricia Mousmanis, MD, CCFP, FCFP, Richmond Hill, ON
Marilee A. Nowgesic, SOGC, Ottawa, ON
Andrea Page, FITMOM Toronto, ON
Andrea L. Rideout, MS, CCGC, CGC Halifax, NS
Anne Roggensack, MD, Calgary, AB
Alyson Shaw, MD, FRCPC, Ottawa, ON
Geneviève St-Gelais, SOGC, Ottawa, ON
Marie-Soleil Wagner, MD, MSc, FRCSC, Montréal, QC
R. Douglas Wilson, MD, University of Calgary, Calgary, AB
Jennifer Wood, Edmonton, AB
Natalie Wright, SOGC, Ottawa, ON
Mark H. Yudin, MD, Toronto, ON

Foreword

Pregnancy is a special time in a woman's life as she prepares for the life-changing event of adding a new member to the family. The 4th edition of *Healthy Beginnings* was revised by the Society of Obstetricians and Gynaecologists of Canada to help women have healthier pregnancies.

As in the past, this handbook is for women with low risk pregnancies—about 90% of all pregnancies in Canada. Reducing risk is a key part of having a healthy pregnancy. In this new edition of the handbook, we place greater emphasis on preconception—the time just before the baby is conceived—and also on early pregnancy—the first three months after conception.

The advice and information you will find in *Healthy Beginnings* is "evidence-based." This means that the content reflects current knowledge and comes from the latest proven research and professional practices in Canada. All of the guidelines for care before pregnancy, during pregnancy, and post-partum contained in this handbook have been updated as needed. The information should not be seen as dictating an exclusive course of treatment or procedure to be followed. Your health-care provider should be consulted and will advise you on your pregnancy and/or specific problems.

International research shows that if pregnant women are aware of how their body prepares for birth, what their growing baby needs, as well as the possible problems they may encounter, and how they can be prevented, mothers will have healthier pregnancies and more babies will be born full-size, full-term, and healthy.

Healthy Beginnings provides you with the information you need to make healthy choices during your pregnancy. It serves as a notebook where you can record the details of your pregnancy, prenatal visits, and your birth experience. Forms are included where you can gather important information you will need during your pregnancy. Space has been provided at the end of each chapter for you to write out questions for your next appointments. Combined with the standard records kept by your health-care provider, it will give you a detailed medical record of your pregnancy. Record the changes in your body and your feelings for reference at your next appointment, or even months and years later, when your notes will remind you of this special time.

Enjoy your pregnancy and look forward to meeting your baby!

Nan Schuurmans, MD, FRCSC
Author

Notes to the reader:
In this handbook, masculine and feminine pronouns are used interchangeably for equal representation. The term "health-care provider" is used to refer to obstetricians, gynaecologists, family physicians, nurses, midwives, and other health-care practitioners.

The Baby-Friendly Initiative is a program of the World Health Organization and UNICEF to increase hospital and community support for promoting, supporting, and protecting breastfeeding. The 4th edition of *Healthy Beginnings* complies with the International Code of Marketing of Breast Milk Substitutes and it meets Baby-Friendly Initiative criteria (Practice Outcome Indicators for: Baby-Friendly Hospitals (The Ten Steps), Baby-Friendly Community Health Services (The Seven Points), Appendix 6: Breastfeeding Education Materials for Families). For more information: www.breastfeeding canada.ca/html/bfi.html.

CHAPTER ONE

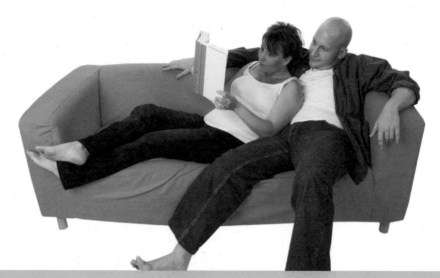

Planning a healthy pregnancy

Almost every woman's menstrual cycle (the time from the first day of the menstrual period to the first day of the next period) varies slightly from month to month. The average length is 28 days but it can range from 21 to 36 days and often changes with age.

Hormones produced by your body control the changes that occur throughout the cycle. Hormones cause an egg to mature in the ovary and they control when the mature egg will be released into your body (ovulation). Ovulation starts about 14 days before your next period.

Introduction

Preconception—the time just before the baby is conceived—and **Early Pregnancy**—the first three months after conception—are now known to be important times when you can reduce risks to you and your baby by making healthy choices.

Most women understand how important it is to take good care of themselves and their unborn child once they are pregnant. What you may not realize is that the healthy choices you and your partner make before conception will also make a difference to you and your unborn child.

Without trying to alarm you, you should be aware that damage to the fetus can occur in the early weeks of pregnancy—before you have missed your period and before you know that you are pregnant. If you are sexually active, there is always a risk that you might get pregnant. Almost half of all pregnancies are not planned. You need to know your body and be prepared for a possible pregnancy. On the other hand, if you are planning a pregnancy, knowing your body will help you become pregnant, as well as help you plan a healthy and risk-free pregnancy.

In this chapter, we'll look at:

• how your body changes in the early stages of pregnancy,
• what you can do to improve your chances of having a healthy pregnancy and a healthy baby—even before conception takes place, and
• how to avoid hazards that may harm you and your baby.

It all begins with an egg

At a certain time during a woman's monthly menstrual cycle, an egg is released from an ovary. This is called *ovulation*. The egg then begins to move down the fallopian tube toward the uterus. If a sperm enters the egg, *fertilization* takes place. The fertilized egg becomes an *embryo*, which begins to grow immediately.

The embryo continues to move down the fallopian tube to the uterus. This takes about seven days. When it reaches the uterus, the embryo attaches to the thickened lining of the uterus (the endometrium). This is called *implantation*.

For the first eight weeks, the fertilized egg is called an *embryo*. After eight weeks, and until birth, the embryo is called a *fetus*.

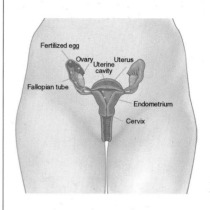

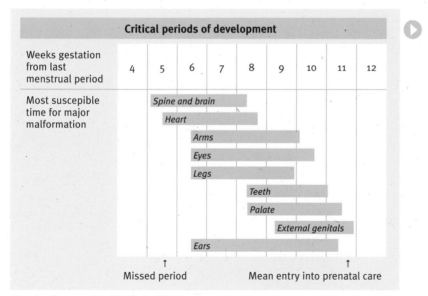

Critical periods of development									
Weeks gestation from last menstrual period	4	5	6	7	8	9	10	11	12
Most suscepible time for major malformation		Spine and brain							
		Heart							
			Arms						
			Eyes						
			Legs						
					Teeth				
					Palate				
							External genitals		
			Ears						

↑ Missed period   ↑ Mean entry into prenatal care

Reproduced by permission of the March of Dimes.

The time when a fetus is most likely to be harmed during pregnancy is also the time when many women may not know they are pregnant. This is between 17 and 56 days after conception, or 4 to 10 weeks from your last menstrual period. At this time, alcohol, or a lack of vital nutrients, particularly folic acid, can cause serious harm to the fetus.

How your body supports new life

During the nine months you are pregnant, your body will provide your baby with everything it needs to live and grow. The uterus protects the fetus in a sac filled with liquid (amniotic fluid). All the nutrients and oxygen the fetus needs will come from the **placenta**, an organ that begins to develop where the embryo is implanted in your uterus. The placenta is made up of blood vessels and tissue. It is firmly attached to the lining of your uterus and continues to grow throughout your pregnancy.

The **umbilical cord** is the lifeline that links your baby to the placenta and to you. The placenta is like a trading post for the blood supply passing between you and your baby. It's where nutrients, oxygen, and protective antibodies travel from your blood to your baby's blood. On the return trip, fetal waste travels from your baby's blood into your bloodstream and is removed by your organs.

The placenta also produces hormones, such as estrogen and progesterone. These hormones cause many of the changes that occur in your body

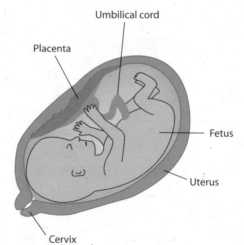

Fetal environment

during pregnancy. One of the most important hormones, which only the placenta can produce, is called human chorionic gonadotrophin (HCG). When you take a pregnancy test, the test tells you whether or not this hormone is in your urine or blood. If it is, you are pregnant!

Visit your health-care provider before you get pregnant

If you are planning a pregnancy, make an appointment for a check-up with your health-care provider. The purpose of this visit is to make sure you are in good health and that your lifestyle will support a healthy baby.

TIPS FOR WHEN YOU VISIT YOUR HEALTH-CARE PROVIDER

Every time you see your health-care provider, consult these tips. They will help you be organized and feel comfortable.

- *BEFORE your appointment, write down your questions and any details you want to share. Ask your partner, a family member, or a friend to come with you. Two sets of ears are always better than one.*

- *DURING your appointment, ask for a clear answer when you did not really understand what was said. Write things down and keep notes. Or ask your partner or friend to take notes for you.*

- *BEFORE you leave your appointment, check that you have asked all the questions on your list and that you understood what your health-care provider was telling you. Make sure you know what will happen next, when your next appointment will be, and if there are any tests that you need to take. Make sure you know who to contact if you have any problems or questions.*

- *AFTER your appointment, write down what you discussed and what happens next. Keep your notes.*

Adapted from the U.K. National Health Service's leaflet "Questions to ask."

I DON'T HAVE TO MENTION THAT, DO I?

When you are talking about your health, and your baby's health, be direct and fully honest about your history and lifestyle.

Your health-care team needs to see the whole picture to help you plan for a healthy pregnancy and birth.

DO YOU HAVE A HEALTH-CARE PROVIDER?

Regular health care is important during pregnancy. If you live in a rural or remote community, you might have limited access to prenatal care. Now is a good time to contact your local health centre, clinic, or nursing station to discuss what is available. Doing so will help you and your future baby get the best care possible.

- *You missed your period.*

- *You feel more tired than usual.*

- *Your breasts feel tingly or tender.*

- *You need to urinate often.*

- *You feel bloated.*

- *You feel nauseous (morning sickness).*

- *You have unusual bleeding (different from your normal period).*

Any one of these signs, combined with a missed period, could mean you are pregnant (even if you have been using a reliable form of birth control).

Be prepared to give honest answers about your medical history, your family, any medications you may take, your diet, your past pregnancies, your sexual history, and the kind of work you do. Your health and your baby's health may depend on this important information. If you are in good health, you probably won't need to see your health-care provider again until you suspect you are pregnant.

Learn about pregnancy

When you are planning to start or add to your family, you need to learn what to expect during pregnancy and how to prepare for childbirth. This is also a good time to learn about breastfeeding. Studies show that women who learn about pregnancy are the ones most likely to have a more positive childbirth experience. Your health-care provider and prenatal classes are good sources of information, and women in the study said that what they learned helped them to be more in control throughout their pregnancy and in childbirth. They also felt more fulfilled during the experience.

- In one study, women who received prenatal education needed less medicine to control pain during labour. This suggests they either had less pain or they knew how to cope better with the pain they had.
- Another study showed that women were more likely to carry their babies to full term when they knew about the kinds of risk factors that can cause a preterm birth (see page 77).

As you plan, remember that you play an important role in having a healthy pregnancy and a healthy baby. Regular prenatal care and keeping yourself healthy and informed are excellent steps to give your baby a healthy beginning.

WOMEN AGED 35 AND OLDER

Most women aged 35 and older will have a healthy pregnancy and a healthy baby. But some women in this age group are also more likely to have certain difficulties when they are pregnant. They may need to take special precautions. If you are in this age group, you should be aware that:

• it may take longer to become pregnant,

• you may have twins or triplets (a multiple birth),

• your baby could be born with a chromosome difference,

• you may get diabetes when you are pregnant,

• you may have high blood pressure when you are pregnant.

Talk to your health-care provider about how you can work together to have the healthiest pregnancy possible.

To learn more about pregnancy for women aged 35 and older, visit the Best Start Resource Centre website at www.beststart.org/resources/rep_health/index.html.

Your medical history

Some past or current health problems can affect the outcome of your pregnancy. Women who have serious medical conditions—such as heart disease, diabetes, or high blood pressure—may need to be followed closely throughout pregnancy by a specialist in that field. Women who are overweight should be tested for diabetes. If you have epilepsy, your neurologist should review your medications before you get pregnant.

MY MEDICAL HISTORY

Check all problems and conditions, and list all operations, that apply to you:

☐ *Problems with an anaesthetic*

☐ *Operations*

List all operations:

_____

_____

☐ *Blood transfusion in the year ____*

☐ *High cholesterol*

☐ *Problems with my heart*

☐ *High blood pressure*

☐ *Diabetes*

☐ *Problems with blood clots in my legs or in my lungs*

☐ *An illness that causes seizures (such as epilepsy)*

☐ *Problems with my kidneys or bladder*

☐ *A serious infection that requires me to take medication*

List of all infectious diseases you have had:

_____

_____

☐ *A history of mental health problems*

☐ *Problems getting pregnant*

☐ *Allergies*

7

MY FAMILY'S MEDICAL HISTORY

List anyone in your close family—such as your parents, brothers, sisters, and children—who has or has had any of these medical conditions:

Diabetes:

A condition that is passed from parent to child (hereditary):

High blood pressure:

A birth defect:

The birth of twins, triplets, or more:

Other problems you think may be serious:

If you, your partner, or a close relative has a type of disease that is common in your family—such as muscular dystrophy, hemophilia, cystic fibrosis, Tay-Sachs disease, or beta-thalassemia—talk to your health-care provider. You may need to be referred to a geneticist (a specialist in the field of heredity).

Are you overweight?

A healthy body weight promotes good health, lowers your risk of disease, and has important and positive effects on any woman's pregnancy. Being overweight—depending on the degree—can create serious health problems and is linked with many complications in pregnancy. These problems may affect both the baby and the mother.

If you are planning to get pregnant and you are concerned that you may be overweight, you should consult your health-care provider. Women with healthy eating and exercise patterns before pregnancy enjoy reduced

Risks of Being Overweight

Risks for the mother	Risks for the baby
Infertility	Stillbirth
Miscarriage	Birth defects
Early labour and birth (preterm birth)	Needing to stay in hospital after birth (intensive care)
Diabetes	Grows too big (causing problems during birth)
High blood pressure	
Needing to have a C-section (Caesarean section for the birth)	

risks for both themselves and the fetus when they are pregnant. You will also improve your long-term health. Ask your health-care provider to refer you to a dietitian or to suggest an accepted weight-loss program so you can learn about the right amount of food to eat.

Regular exercise is also a key part of losing weight. Guidelines show that people need at least 30 minutes of moderate exercise (that makes you sweat), 5 days a week to enjoy long-term good health. Making changes **before** you get pregnant will help to ensure you have a healthy diet and good exercise habits during pregnancy.

Medicines and pregnancy

Almost all medicines you take may cross through the placenta into a growing baby's body. This includes both prescription and non-prescription medicines. Remember, you share what goes into your body with your baby.

While not many medicines are proven to be harmful to a growing baby, there has not been much research in this area and we do not really know what effect some drugs might have. Drugs that are known to cause harm usually do so within the first few weeks of pregnancy—when the baby's major body systems are still forming. If you are taking medicines of any kind, it is best to review them with your health-care provider before you become pregnant. It is best to avoid non-prescription drugs, including herbal products, while you are trying to conceive and during pregnancy. Talk to your health-care provider before you use any kind of drug, herb, plant, or home remedy. They will know or find out how safe these products are for pregnant women.

If you would like to know more about toxic substances that may harm your baby, talk to the team at the Motherisk Program at the Hospital for Sick Children in Toronto by calling 1-416-813-6780. Or visit their website at www.motherisk.org.

If you are planning a pregnancy and are taking prescription medicines for a health problem, it is very important that you discuss your options

---

WHAT PRESCRIPTION AND NON-PRESCRIPTION DRUGS, HERBS, AND VITAMINS DO YOU TAKE?

DRUG, HERB, OR VITAMIN
name:

amount you take:

how often you take it:

how long you have been taking it:

DRUG, HERB, OR VITAMIN
name:

amount you take:

how often you take it:

how long you have been taking it:

DRUG, HERB, OR VITAMIN
name:

amount you take:

how often you take it:

how long you have been taking it:

with your health-care provider before you get pregnant. Two common prescription drugs that may be hazardous to the baby are:

- coumadin (a blood thinner), and
- drugs to control epilepsy.

If you are taking a drug that is known to harm the baby, you may need to change to a drug that will still give you the treatment you need and is also deemed safe to use during pregnancy. If the prescription cannot be changed, your health-care provider may advise you to reduce your dosage or to stop using the drug during your pregnancy, if it is safe to do so.

Immunizations and infections

When you are planning your pregnancy, it's a good time to check whether all your immunizations are up-to-date. Infections you can prevent, such as rubella, can harm your unborn baby. In other cases, the vaccines themselves can harm an embryo when a pregnant woman receives them. It's best to get all your immunizations up-to-date before you become pregnant, and then to wait at least three months before you conceive. If your immunizations are not up-to-date and you become pregnant, talk to your health-care provider.

A general rule is that pregnant women should not get "live virus" vaccines—those made from weak versions of the infection. Examples of "live virus" vaccines include: measles, mumps, and rubella. Vaccines made from dead viruses (or toxoids)—such as the influenza and tetanus vaccines—are safe. If you are unsure about a vaccine, ask your health-care provider.

If your job, lifestyle, or health history makes you more likely to come into contact with illness, your health-care provider may recommend that you get other vaccines, such as the hepatitis B vaccine.

The Public Health Agency of Canada provides a guide about immunization for pregnant and breastfeeding women. It is available at www.phac-aspc.gc.ca.

Lifestyle and sexual history

You may not feel comfortable talking about your sexual habits. But as with drug use, your health-care provider asks these questions to help reduce risks to your baby.

If you have ever had sex without using a condom—especially if you have had more than one sexual partner—you may have been exposed to a **sexually transmitted infection** such as genital herpes, genital warts, chlamydia, gonorrhea, syphilis, or the HIV virus (which causes AIDS).

Some sexually transmitted infections (STIs) can be cured. Others cannot. Some need to be treated to reduce the risk of infecting the baby at birth.

- Based on your lifestyle and sexual history, certain tests can help you plan your prenatal care.
- HIV testing is offered to all women who are pregnant or are thinking about getting pregnant. The reason? An effective treatment exists. It can greatly reduce the chance that a woman who is HIV-positive will give the virus to her baby.
- Women who live with a disease that comes back again and again— such as genital herpes or genital warts—can still have a normal pregnancy. Sometimes, particularly around the time of the baby's birth, these mothers may need special care.

To learn more about STIs, visit www.sexualityandu.ca.

If you have been pregnant before

Your health-care provider will ask you about your past pregnancies and about any problems you may have had during the pregnancy, during labour and delivery, and after giving birth. Knowing about any previous

---

**HIV IN PREGNANCY
TOLL-FREE HELP LINE
1-888-246-5840**

Motherisk's toll-free HIV Healthline offers private advice to Canadian women, their families, and health-care providers about the risks of HIV (the human immunodeficiency virus) and HIV treatment in pregnancy. Motherisk also helps HIV specialists and community groups across Canada work together to assess the risks and safety of different HIV treatments.

1. *A rise in hormone levels changes the lining of the uterus so it is ready to receive the embryo.*

2. *The ovary releases an egg (ovulation) about 14 days before the next period begins.*

3. *Discharge from your vagina at the time of ovulation becomes more plentiful and clear.*

4. *Your body temperature rises for a few days just after ovulation.*

5. *You may feel mild cramps in your lower abdomen or bloating near the time of ovulation.*

problems will alert your health-care provider to any possible problems now. This can help to prevent them from happening again. Even if you have had problems in the past, you can still have a normal, healthy pregnancy. It's always very important to tell your health-care provider as many details as possible about your health, so that both of you can plan for any special care you might need.

I have been pregnant before			
	1st	2nd	3rd
Date:			
Name of hospital:			
Hours in labour:			
Type of delivery (normal, forceps, C-section):			
Complications:			
Baby was boy or girl:			
Baby's birth weight:			
Other pregnancies (miscarriages and/or therapeutic abortions):			

Keep track of your monthly cycle

If you are not yet pregnant, now is a good time to start keeping a record of your menstrual cycle. If you are already pregnant, well . . . you could suggest that your friends do so!

A cycle starts on the first day of your period. It ends on the first day of your next period. Then it begins all over again. You can use a calendar to track your cycle. This will help you to predict your next period, know what is normal for you, and figure out when you are most fertile (most likely to conceive). Once you become pregnant, your knowledge of your body's cycles will help your health-care provider calculate your **due date**—the day your baby is expected to be born. Your due date and the date of your last menstrual period will also help measure how your baby is growing throughout your pregnancy.

How easy it will be for you to become pregnant depends a great deal on your menstrual cycle. You are most fertile near the time of ovulation. So, if you hope to get pregnant, you and your partner will want to have sexual intercourse around that time. But how can you tell when you are ovulating? The easiest way to tell is to count back 14 days from the day when you predict your next period will start. Most women do not have to do anything else to get pregnant. It just happens naturally.

If you need to be more certain of the best days to try to get pregnant, watch for changes in your body that signal ovulation.

What if I am using the "pill", the "patch", or the "ring"?

If you are using hormonal birth control—such as oral contraceptives (the "pill"), the transdermal patch (the "patch"), or the vaginal ring (the "ring")—you should allow yourself at least one normal menstrual cycle before you try to become pregnant. Taking a rest will allow your body to return to its own natural pace. To protect yourself from pregnancy during this rest period, use a condom. If you become pregnant while taking hormonal birth control, stop immediately. But don't worry, there are no known ill effects to the baby if you become pregnant.

example:

FEBRUARY

S	M	T	W	T	F	S
			1	2	3	4
5	6	7	8	9	10	11
12	13	14	15	16	17	18
19	20	(21)	(22)	(23)	(24)	(25)
26	27	28				

This chart shows that the first day of this woman's last menstrual period was February 21.

What about other forms of birth control?

If you use an injectable contraceptive (the "shot")—a birth control method that is injected into your body—you should wait at least six to nine months after your last injection before you try to become pregnant. It takes an average of nine months for your fertility to return after your last injection. You may still become pregnant before nine months pass.

If you use spermicidal foams, jellies, condoms, or a diaphragm, you do not have to wait a full cycle before trying to become pregnant. You can start immediately.

If you are using an intrauterine device (IUD) for birth control, you should have it removed before you try to get pregnant. It is best to wait until you have at least one normal period after the IUD is removed before you try to get pregnant. If you have an IUD in place and you suspect you may be pregnant, visit your health-care provider for a pregnancy test. If you do get pregnant with an IUD in place, you should have it removed. It can cause a miscarriage, infection, or preterm birth.

What about nutrition?

Eating well before you become pregnant will help prepare your body to meet the nutritional needs of your developing baby when you do conceive. Follow *Eating Well with Canada's Food Guide* (see pages 17 and 18), both before and during your pregnancy.

- It promotes a wide variety of healthy foods you should eat every day.
- It provides tips and advice for women at all ages and stages of life—such as women who are pregnant, are breastfeeding, or are of childbearing age.

By setting good eating habits now, you are also likely to find it easier to keep eating well throughout your pregnancy. For most healthy women, following the guide will ensure that you get enough of the vitamins, minerals, and other nutrients you need for a healthy pregnancy. In addition to eating a healthy, balanced diet, pregnant women should also eat often. It's important for pregnant women to avoid long periods without eating (more than 12 hours) to support a healthy pregnancy. The best approach is for pregnant women to eat three meals and three small snacks spread throughout each day.

If you have special nutritional needs (see list in sidebar on pages 15 and 16), get support from your health-care provider who may suggest that you get help from a dietitian.

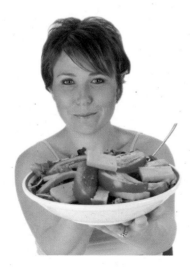

NUTRITION QUIZ

As you read this list, check off any statements that are true for you.

☐ *I am on a diet to lose weight.*

☐ *I sometimes "fast" or skip meals.*

☐ *I do very strenuous exercise.*

☐ *I weigh too much (overweight).*

☐ *I weigh too little (underweight).*

☐ *I have an eating disorder.*

☐ *I do not consume enough milk products.*

☐ *I have food allergies.*

☐ *I am a vegetarian.*

☐ *I have a history of low iron in my blood (anemia).*

☐ *I am expecting twins or multiple births.*

☐ *I gave birth to a low birth weight baby in the past (less than 5 lbs 8 oz/2.5 kg).*

☐ *I am under 18 years old.*

☐ *I have diabetes.*

☐ *I have a serious illness that affects what I can eat.*

(Continued)

NUTRITION QUIZ (CONTINUED)

☐ I am under a lot of stress and it affects my food intake.

☐ I suffer from serious vomiting problems.

☐ I do not have enough money to buy the food I need.

☐ I have high cholesterol.

☐ I am always constipated (cannot have a bowel movement).

☐ I do not eat fish.

☐ I do not eat red meat.

If you checked off any of these boxes, then you have special nutritional needs that you should discuss with your health-care provider.

MAKING HEALTHY FOOD CHOICES

Do you want to know what's in the food you just bought? Healthy Eating is in Store for You™ will help you learn how to read and use the nutrition labels on food that comes in packages. This guide is sponsored by the Canadian Diabetes Association and Dietitians of Canada. Visit the website at www.healthyeatingisinstore.ca.

Different people need different amounts of food

The number of servings (from the four food groups) that people need on a daily basis is different depending on your age and whether you are male or female. The recommended number of Food Guide servings is an average amount that people should try to eat each day. Pregnant and breastfeeding women need a few more calories. For most women, this means eating an extra two or three Food Guide servings from any of the food groups each day in addition to their recommended number of Food Guide servings per day.

How can you get these extra Food Guide servings? Have them as a snack, or add them to your usual meals. For instance, instead of having an extra snack made up of two Food Guide servings, you may choose to have one extra Food Guide serving of vegetable or fruit at breakfast and one extra Food Guide serving of milk and alternatives at supper.

Canada's Food Guide is available in these languages: English, French, Arabic, Chinese, Farsi (Persian), Korean, Punjabi, Russian, Spanish, Tagalog, Tamil, and Urdu. There is also a tailored Food Guide for First Nations, Inuit, and Métis (see page 18).

Eating Well with Canada's Food Guide
Recommended Number of Food Guide Servings per Day—Females ages 19-50

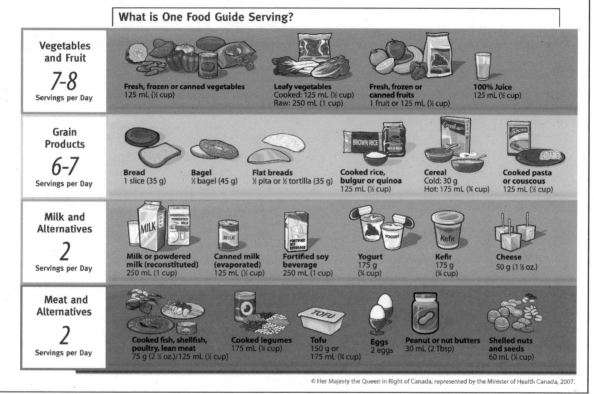

What is One Food Guide Serving?

Vegetables and Fruit
7-8
Servings per Day

- **Fresh, frozen or canned vegetables** 125 mL (½ cup)
- **Leafy vegetables** Cooked: 125 mL (½ cup) Raw: 250 mL (1 cup)
- **Fresh, frozen or canned fruits** 1 fruit or 125 mL (½ cup)
- **100% Juice** 125 mL (½ cup)

Grain Products
6-7
Servings per Day

- **Bread** 1 slice (35 g)
- **Bagel** ½ bagel (45 g)
- **Flat breads** ½ pita or ½ tortilla (35 g)
- **Cooked rice, bulgur or quinoa** 125 mL (½ cup)
- **Cereal** Cold: 30 g Hot: 175 mL (¾ cup)
- **Cooked pasta or couscous** 125 mL (½ cup)

Milk and Alternatives
2
Servings per Day

- **Milk or powdered milk (reconstituted)** 250 mL (1 cup)
- **Canned milk (evaporated)** 125 mL (½ cup)
- **Fortified soy beverage** 250 mL (1 cup)
- **Yogurt** 175 g (¾ cup)
- **Kefir** 175 g (¾ cup)
- **Cheese** 50 g (1 ½ oz.)

Meat and Alternatives
2
Servings per Day

- **Cooked fish, shellfish, poultry, lean meat** 75 g (2 ½ oz.)/125 mL (½ cup)
- **Cooked legumes** 175 mL (¾ cup)
- **Tofu** 150 g or 175 mL (¾ cup)
- **Eggs** 2 eggs
- **Peanut or nut butters** 30 mL (2 Tbsp)
- **Shelled nuts and seeds** 60 mL (¼ cup)

© Her Majesty the Queen in Right of Canada, represented by the Minister of Health Canada, 2007.

Source: Eating Well with Canada's Food Guide (2007), Health Canada. Reproduced with the permission of the Minister of Public Works and Government Services Canada, 2008.
www.hc.sc.gc.ca/fn-an/food-guide-aliment/index_e.html

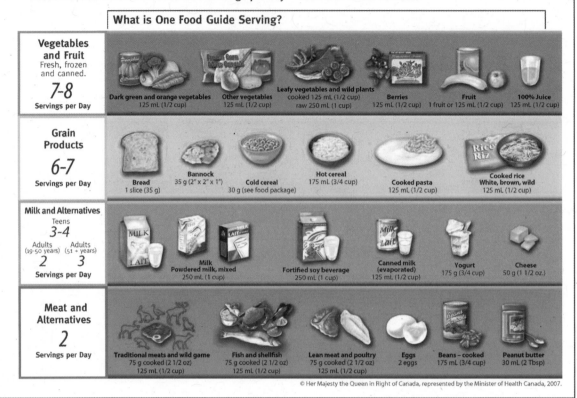

Eating Well with Canada's Food Guide—First Nations, Inuit and Métis
Recommended Number of Food Guide Servings per Day—Teen and Adult Females

© Her Majesty the Queen in Right of Canada, represented by the Minister of Health Canada, 2007.

Source: Eating Well with Canada's Food Guide – First Nations, Inuit and Métis (2007), Health Canada. Reproduced with the permission of the Minister of Public Works and Government Services Canada, 2008. www.hc-sc.gc.ca/fn-an/food-guide-aliment/index_e.html

Guidelines from Health Canada

Vegetables and fruit:

Eat at least one dark green (such as broccoli or spinach) and one orange (such as carrots or sweet potatoes) vegetable each day.

Choose vegetables and fruit prepared with little or no added fat, sugar, or salt. Enjoy vegetables steamed, baked, or stir-fried instead of deep-fried.

Grain products:

Ensure that at least half your daily grain products are whole grain.

Include bread, pasta, rice, cereal, and other grains, such as barley, oats, and quinoa.

Enjoy whole-grain breads, oatmeal, or whole-wheat pasta.

Choose grain products that are low in fat, sugar, or salt. Compare products and make wise choices by reading the Nutrition Facts label.

Milk and alternatives:

Have 500 ml (two cups) of 2%, 1%, or skim milk every day.

Drink fortified soy beverages if you do not drink milk.

Select lower fat milk alternatives. Compare the Nutrition Facts label on yogurts or cheeses to help make wise choices.

Meat and alternatives:

Have meat alternatives, such as beans, lentils, and tofu, as often as possible.

Select lean meat and alternatives prepared with little or no added fat or salt.

IF IT COSTS TOO MUCH TO EAT WELL

Some women are not always able to afford the food they need to have a healthy pregnancy and baby. Talk to your health-care provider or community health nurse about food programs in your community.

The Canadian government provides funding to community groups to support the food needs of pregnant women at risk. A program in your community may be able to provide you with the support you need. To learn more about the Canada Prenatal Nutrition Program, visit the Public Health Agency of Canada's website at: www.phac-aspc.gc.ca/dca-dea/ programs-mes/cpnp_main-eng.php.

Trim the visible fat from meats and remove the skin from poultry. Use cooking methods such as roasting, baking, or poaching that require little, or no added fat.

Include at least two Food Guide servings of fish each week (see list of fish on pages 21 and 22).

Unsaturated fat:

For good health, include a small amount (30–45 ml or 2–3 tablespoons) of unsaturated fat each day. This amount includes oil used for cooking, salad dressings, margarine, and mayonnaise. Unsaturated vegetable oils include: canola, corn, flaxseed, olive, peanut, soybean, and sunflower. Limit butter, hard margarine, lard, and shortening.

Foods to limit or avoid during pregnancy

Foods that may contain bacteria

Foods that contain bacteria and parasites are very risky for pregnant women and their unborn children. Listeriosis is a rare but serious disease. It can cause miscarriage, stillbirth, illness in the mother, and severe illness in the newborn. Toxoplasmosis can also cause infection. The effects on the mother may be mild but it can cause birth defects in the baby.

To prevent infections from food, pregnant women should avoid the following:

- raw fish, especially shellfish such as oysters and clams
- undercooked meat, poultry, and seafood (for example, hot dogs, non-dried deli-meats, refrigerated pâté, meat spreads, and refrigerated smoked seafood and fish)
- all foods made with raw or lightly cooked eggs (for example, homemade Caesar vinaigrette)

Common things to avoid or limit when you are pregnant

Alcohol
Avoid it. Do not drink any kind of alcohol in any amount.

Caffeine
Limit yourself to less than 1 or 2 cups of coffee each day (300 mg/day).

Herbal teas
- *Some teas are safe if you drink only 2 or 3 cups a day. They are: citrus peel, ginger, lemon, orange, and rose hip.*
- *Other teas are not safe. Do not drink herbal teas that contain chamomile, aloe, coltsfoot, juniper berries, pennyroyal, buckthorn bark, comfrey, labrador tea, sassafras, duck roots, lobelia, or senna.*

Artificial sweeteners
Aspartame is the most common one. It has not been proven to be a risk. Products containing artificial sweeteners should not be used in place of nutrient-rich foods.

- unpasteurized milk products and foods made from them, including soft and semi-soft cheeses such as Brie or Camembert
- unpasteurized juices, such as unpasteurized apple cider
- raw sprouts, especially alfalfa sprouts

Do not store fresh or cooked meat or poultry (in the refrigerator) for longer than 2 or 3 days. Keep uncooked meats separate from other foods; wash hands, cooking utensils, and cooking surfaces well after handling uncooked meat; and wash raw vegetables (especially pre-cut and ready-to-eat vegetables) thoroughly before eating.

Important facts about fish

Fish is an especially important food in pregnancy because it is a good source of protein and omega-3 fatty acids. There is evidence that regular consumption of fish by pregnant women and women who may become pregnant plays a role in normal fetal brain and eye development. Canada's Food Guide recommends eating at least 150 grams (2 Food Guide servings) of fish each week.

Some types of fish have higher levels of beneficial fatty acids than others. Fish and shellfish that contain higher levels of these fatty acids and are also low in mercury include:

- anchovy
- capelin
- char
- hake
- herring
- Atlantic mackerel
- mullet
- pollock (Boston bluefish)
- salmon

Fish is an excellent source of protein and omega-3 fatty acids. Both are very important for your baby's growth and development. Check this section (pages 21 and 22) for a list of fish to choose more often.

- smelt
- rainbow trout
- lake whitefish
- blue crab
- shrimp

Some types of fish contain higher levels of mercury than others. Mercury in fish may hinder brain development in your baby. You need to limit your intake of the kinds of fish that are known to have high mercury content to no more than 150 grams or 2 Food Guide servings per month.

Women who are trying to get pregnant, or who are pregnant or breastfeeding, should limit consumption to 150 grams per month of the following fish:

- fresh or frozen tuna
- shark
- swordfish
- marlin
- orange roughy
- escolar

They should also limit consumption of canned Albacore "white" tuna (does not apply to canned light tuna) to 300 grams a week. Canned Albacore tuna is also often called canned white tuna. It is not the same as canned light tuna. Canned light tuna contains other species of tuna such as skipjack, yellowfin, and tongol, which are relatively low in mercury.

For up-to-date warnings about fish consumption across Canada, see Environment Canada's website at www.ec.gc.ca/MERCURY/EN/fc.cfm.

For more details on foods to avoid during pregnancy, see the Government of Ontario's Healthy Ontario website at www.healthyontario.com/FeatureDetails.aspx?feature_id=4078.

Other healthy and essential nutrients

Omega-3 fatty acids

These types of fats are considered "healthy" (your body needs them and so does your baby) and "essential" because your body cannot make them by itself. You must get omega-3 fatty acids through the food you eat (refer to sidebar *Food sources of omega-3 fatty acids* list). Omega-3 fatty acids have been linked to health benefits for your heart, your joints, and your mental health. They have also been linked to better blood flow to the placenta and the growing baby, and they may help to prevent preterm labour. In a growing baby, these fats support good development of the brain and nervous system. They also improve the baby's vision and skin.

Minerals and vitamins

Do I need to take special vitamins?

Prenatal vitamins are multivitamins that are made for pregnant women. All pregnant women should take prenatal vitamins daily. They contain many important and beneficial vitamins and minerals. One of the most important

FOOD SOURCES OF OMEGA-3 FATTY ACIDS

- *salmon and other coldwater fish such as char, herring, mackerel, sardines, and trout*
- *omega-3 fortified eggs*
- *walnut oil*
- *flax oil*
- *vegetable oils such as olive, canola, soybean, and soft (non-hydrogenated) margarine*

is *folic acid.* It will help your baby grow and it will help prevent certain birth defects. Following Canada's Food Guide and taking a prenatal vitamin a day will help you meet your nutrient needs during pregnancy. Depending on how healthy you are and what you eat, you may need to add more calcium, vitamin D, or iron in the form of vitamin pills. Refer to the sections that follow to see if you may need to take special minerals or vitamins while you are pregnant. Extra calcium and iron are better absorbed when you take them between meals and at different times. If you are taking extra iron, ensure that your multivitamin also contains zinc. Your health-care provider can help you determine the vitamins that are right for you.

Calcium and vitamin D

Women who are pregnant or breastfeeding need calcium and vitamin D to maintain bone strength. While she is pregnant, a woman needs both of them to help her body build her baby's skeleton. The recommended daily intake for calcium is 1000 mg/day. For vitamin D, it is 200 IU/day.

Milk and alternatives are at the top of the list of good sources for calcium and vitamin D. They are rich in calcium, and the kind of calcium they contain is well absorbed by the body. Milk and fortified soy beverages are enriched with vitamin D, which also helps you absorb calcium. Other sources of calcium include sardines, salmon (with the bones), bok choy, sesame seeds, nuts, legumes, and broccoli.

Some people may be at risk of poor vitamin D status, particularly if they do not include 2 cups of milk or fortified soy beverages in their diet every day. If you are at risk for low vitamin D or calcium intake, you may want to take vitamin supplements.

Risk factors for low vitamin D levels:

• not drinking milk
• regularly wearing clothing that covers most of your skin
• living in northern parts of the world (most of Canada) during the winter months
• being indoors most of the time
• regularly using sunscreen (greater than SPF 8)
• having dark skin

What about the dangers of too much of a vitamin?

Taking more than the recommended dose of vitamins can be harmful. For example, too much vitamin A (more than 10,000 IU/3,000 mcg RAE per day) is linked to birth defects. Make sure you do not take more than one tablet per day of your multivitamin. Read the label on any vitamins you buy outside a pharmacy. If you have doubts about the amount of a vitamin you are taking, ask your health-care provider before you take it. She may suggest getting further help or advice from a dietitian.

Dietary sources of calcium

	Serving size		Calcium (mg)
MILK AND ALTERNATIVES			
Cheese, parmesan, grated	50 g	(2 oz)	554
Cheese, cheddar	50 g	(2 oz)	360
Ricotta cheese, with partly skimmed milk	125 ml	(1/2 cup)	356
Cheese, brick	50 g	(2 oz)	337
Milk, chocolate flavour, powder, with 2% M.F.	250 ml	(1 cup)	328
Yogurt, plain, 1% to 2% M.F.	175 g	(3/4 cup)	320
Beverage, soy, fluid, enriched	250 ml	(1 cup)	319
Milk, fluid, partly skimmed, 2% M.F.	250 ml	(1 cup)	302
Cheese, mozzarella (52% water, 22.5% M.F.)	50 g	(2 oz)	269
Ice cream, vanilla, 11% M.F.	250 ml	(1 cup)	195
Yogurt, frozen	250 ml	(1 cup)	184
Cheese, cottage, creamed (4.5% M.F.)	125 ml	(1/2 cup)	71
FOOD MADE FROM MILK PRODUCTS			
Milkshake: vanilla, thick	250 ml	(1 cup)	364
Soup: tomato, canned, condensed, whole milk added	250 ml	(1 cup)	168
Pudding, chocolate	125 ml	(1/2 cup)	111
OTHER FOOD SOURCES OF CALCIUM			
Sardine, Atlantic, canned with oil, drained solids with bone	75 g		286
Salmon, pink, canned, drained solids with bone	75 g		208
Tofu (made with calcium sulfate)	150 g		1442
Seeds: sesame seeds, whole, roasted and toasted	40 g	(1/4 cup)	376
LESS IMPORTANT SOURCES OF CALCIUM			
Kale, frozen, boiled, drained	125 ml	(1/2 cup)	95
Cabbage, Chinese (pak-choi, bok choy), boiled, drained	125 ml	(1/2 cup)	84
Orange, Florida, raw	1 fruit (7 cm dia)		65
Nuts, almonds, dried, blanched	25 g	(1/4 cup)	52
Broccoli, frozen, chopped, unprepared	125 ml	(1/2 cup)	46
Beans, lima, canned, solids and liquid	125 ml	(1/2 cup)	37

Source: Health Canada, Canadian Nutrient File, 2007.

Folic acid

Studies have found that the risk of having a baby with neural tube defects (which affect the baby's brain and spinal cord) is lower if women take a daily vitamin that contains folic acid (0.4–1.0 mg) **before they become pregnant and during the early weeks of pregnancy.**

Folic acid is a vitamin that helps prevent **neural tube birth defects** (NTDs). It may also prevent other birth defects.

NTDs occur when a baby's spinal cord, skull, or brain does not develop normally between the third and the fourth week of pregnancy. During this time, many women do not even know they are pregnant.

Women who eat well and take a daily multivitamin that contains 0.4–1.0 milligram (mg) of folic acid each day during the three months before they become pregnant—and throughout pregnancy—can reduce their risk of having a baby with an NTD.

Women who may be at higher risk (see sidebar) may benefit from taking a higher dose of folic acid—as much as 5 mg per day. You should discuss this with your health-care provider.

Food sources of folic acid

(based on usual serving size)

EXCELLENT SOURCES OF FOLIC ACID
55 μG (MICROGRAMS) OR MORE

Cooked beans (fava, kidney, pinto, roman, soy, and white), chickpeas, lentils
Cooked spinach, asparagus
Romaine lettuce
Orange juice, canned pineapple juice
Sunflower seeds

GOOD SOURCES OF FOLIC ACID
33 μG (MICROGRAMS) OR MORE

Cooked lima beans, corn, broccoli, green peas, brussels sprouts, beets
Bean sprouts
Oranges
Honeydew melon
Raspberries, blackberries
Avocado
Roasted peanuts
Wheat germ

OTHER SOURCES OF FOLIC ACID
11 μG (MICROGRAMS) OR MORE

Cooked carrots, beet greens, sweet potato, snow peas, summer and winter squash, rutabaga, cabbage, green beans
Cashews, roasted peanuts, walnuts
Eggs
Strawberries, banana, grapefruit, cantaloupe
Whole wheat or white bread
Pork, kidney
Breakfast cereals
Milk, all types

FOLIC ACID QUIZ

Do you need extra folic acid while you are pregnant? Read the list below and check off any statements that are true for you.

☐ *I have epilepsy.*

☐ *I have anemia.*

☐ *I have diabetes that requires me to take insulin.*

☐ *I or my partner had a pregnancy in which the baby had a* **congenital anomaly** *(see sidebar on page 28).*

☐ *I or my partner have a close relative who was born with a* **congenital anomaly** *(see sidebar on page 28).*

☐ *I use alcohol or recreational drugs (see pages 32 and 33).*

☐ *I do not eat healthy foods each day (see page 14).*

☐ *I am obese (see page 8).*

If you are planning a pregnancy and you checked any of the boxes above, you should talk to your health-care provider about the right amount of folic acid.

They are structural defects that happen while the baby develops during pregnancy. They may affect the baby for life. Some examples are:
- *neural tube defects (anencephaly, meningocele)*
- *facial cleft that affects the mouth*
- *structural heart disease*
- *limb defect*
- *urinary tract anomaly*
- *hydrocephaly*

AM I AT RISK FOR ANEMIA?

As you read this list, check off any of the statements that are true for you.

☐ *I have been told in the past that I have low hemoglobin or anemia.*
☐ *I have a history of heavy bleeding during my periods.*
☐ *I do not eat red meat.*
☐ *I have a chronic illness.*
☐ *I have a family history of anemia.*
☐ *I am very thin (underweight).*
☐ *My planned or current pregnancy is happening very close to a previous pregnancy, or I have had one or more closely spaced pregnancies.*
☐ *I am expecting a multiple birth (twins or more).*

If you checked off any of the boxes above, speak to your health-care provider.

Folic acid and other vitamins are very important to your growing baby's health and development (see "Do I need to take special vitamins?" on page 23). Talk to your health-care provider or community health nurse if you cannot find or buy the vitamins you need.

Note: In Canada, as of November 1998, the law required that folic acid be added to white flour and pasta products labelled "enriched." This adds about 100 µg (0.1 mg) of folic acid to the average woman's diet every day. As well, women who are planning a pregnancy, or are in the early stages of pregnancy, should eat foods rich in folic acid, and take a daily supplement containing folic acid.

What is anemia?

Hemoglobin is a substance found in the blood that carries oxygen from your lungs to other parts of your body and to your growing baby. Anemia means that you have lower levels of hemoglobin in your blood. During pregnancy, a woman may develop anemia because she has low levels of iron in her body. This can affect her energy level, her ability to exercise, and the amount of oxygen her body provides to both her and her baby.

Anemia is common in pregnant women. During pregnancy, your body needs more iron, but it's hard to meet your increased needs through diet alone (see sidebar on page 29). Your health-care provider can perform a blood test to find out if your hemoglobin level is normal (between 110 and 112 g/L). If the level is low, your health-care provider may prescribe an iron supplement that you will need to take along with your prenatal vitamins.

Our bodies absorb iron from animal sources better than iron from non-animal sources. Vitamin C helps your body absorb iron. This means if you have a glass of orange juice (Vitamin C) with your boiled egg (iron), you will be helping your body absorb the iron better.

Nutrition tracking

Use this chart to keep track of your eating habits for one week. Then, compare your habits with the recommendations in *Eating Well with Canada's Food Guide*. Use this as a guide to eating during your pregnancy. Mark an "X" for each serving you have eaten during the day.

	Vegetables & Fruit 7–8 servings	Grain Products 6–7 servings	Milk & Alternatives 2 servings	Meat & Alternatives 2 servings	Additional Servings 2–3 servings
Day 1					
Day 2					
Day 3					
Day 4					
Day 5					
Day 6					
Day 7					

Exercise for pregnant women

Women who are physically fit before pregnancy have fewer aches and pains and more energy during their pregnancy. Do not think you need to be an athlete. Just being active on a regular basis (by walking, swimming, or doing yoga) makes a difference to weight maintenance and general well-being.

Dietary sources of iron

MILLIGRAMS (MG) OF IRON FOUND IN EACH 100-GRAM PORTION

EXCELLENT SOURCES OF IRON
Liver (Even though this is an excellent source, you should eat no more than 75 grams (2 ½ oz) of liver once every 2 weeks if you are pregnant.)

GOOD SOURCES OF IRON
Beef (3.1–3.9 mg), veal (3.2–3.6 mg), shrimp (2.1-3.4 mg)

SOURCES OF IRON
Lamb (2.0 mg), chicken (1.3 mg), pork (1.1 mg)

OTHER SOURCES OF IRON
Egg yolk, legumes, tofu
Dark green vegetables (spinach, broccoli, peas)
Dried fruit
Breakfast cereals enriched with iron

WHY SHOULD YOU QUIT SMOKING?

- *My baby will get more oxygen from me.*

- *My baby will be less likely to have breathing problems after she is born.*

- *My baby will be more likely to be a normal weight when he is born.*

- *My baby will be less likely to be born early.*

- *I will breathe better and have more energy.*

- *I will save money.*

- *I will feel good about myself for making a healthy decision for me and my baby.*

If you have been active for at least six months, ask about whether you may continue your sports or workouts safely. As you move further into your pregnancy and your body naturally changes, you may feel mild aches and pains due to looser joints and shifting of your body weight. It may be a good idea to revise your exercise program every trimester to reduce the risk of falls. You should also ask your health-care provider about limiting high-impact activities. Certain high-risk activities like scuba diving are not recommended.

If you have not been active and would like to begin an activity program, "start low and go slow." Exercise is good for you and your baby and, for almost all pregnant women, it is highly recommended. Try regular brisk walking, swimming, strength training for pregnant women, or other activities that will strengthen your heart and lungs and tone your muscles. If you are not physically active when you become pregnant, it is recommended that you wait until the second trimester to start your program. You can read more about exercise during pregnancy in Chapter Two.

Workplace

Women planning a pregnancy should follow all safety rules if they must work with chemicals, solvents, fumes, or radiation. If you are already pregnant, your health-care provider may advise you to avoid any contact with some of these workplace hazards. See the Motherisk website (www.motherisk.org) for more details about exposure risks at work and at home during pregnancy.

Shift work, doing very demanding physical work, working long hours, and having to commute a long distance can sometimes lead to miscarriage or a small or preterm baby. You can read more about how we define very demanding physical (strenuous) work during pregnancy in Chapter Three.

Smoking

There is a clearly proven link between smoking during pregnancy and small or preterm babies. There is also a great deal of evidence suggesting that second-hand smoke harms infants and children. If you or your partner smoke, an excellent way to prepare for being a parent is to **stop smoking now**.

If you are already pregnant, studies show that if you quit smoking before you reach your 16th week, there is less chance that your baby will be born too early or be too small. Some research says your baby can still benefit greatly even if you quit smoking as late as 32 weeks into your pregnancy. As well, studies show that you can increase your baby's birth weight by drastically reducing how much you smoke during your pregnancy. The best way to proceed, if you are planning to have a baby, is to quit smoking **before** you get pregnant. This way, your baby will enjoy the most health benefits. However, it is important to be aware that there are health benefits to quitting at any time, even after your child is born.

If you do smoke, you need to understand the risks of having a small or preterm baby (see page 81). Unfortunately, some women have incorrect beliefs. They think that:

• the risk is not very big or very important, or
• that having a smaller baby is better because the birth will be easier.

The fact is babies born too early and too small (underweight) have a harder time living outside the womb. They are also more likely to have problems sleeping and eating, and are more likely to get sick if they are exposed to illness. It may be hard for you to quit smoking, but support is available. (See page 69 for ways to relieve stress.)

I CAN QUIT SMOKING!

WHY?

I want to be in the best health for my pregnancy.

I want my baby to have the best chance at being healthy.

HOW?

I will change some of my habits (behaviour patterns).

If I smoke after meals, I will get up after a meal and go for a walk.

If I smoke when I feel stressed, I will call a friend, listen to music, or take a bath.

If I smoke before breakfast, I'll quit this cigarette and wait until after I have eaten.

WHAT ABOUT THE PEOPLE AROUND ME?

I will ask others not to smoke around me.

I will go to non-smoking areas when I go out.

A DANGEROUS MYTH

Someone might tell you that quitting smoking during pregnancy can harm your baby. This is not true! Remember: **Quitting is best!**

Decide to quit, believe you can do it, take steps to change your behaviour, and get help!

*There are many people and programs in your community to help you quit smoking. (**See Chapter 9 to learn about resources to help you quit.**)*

NO THANKS, MY BABY IS TOO YOUNG TO DRINK!

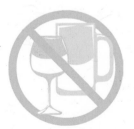

Alcohol

Because of serious health risks, most experts suggest that women avoid all alcohol during their entire pregnancy.

• Alcohol can cause serious brain damage and other health risks for a growing baby. These effects may last a lifetime.
• Babies can suffer cognitive and learning disabilities, developmental conduct and personality disorders, poor growth and development, and facial changes.

How harmful will a mother's drinking be? Mostly, it depends on your own health, how much you drink, and when. The safest choice is not to drink at all during pregnancy.

Alcohol is harmful to my baby

The most well-known result of drinking alcohol during pregnancy is fetal alcohol spectrum disorder (FASD). It is a group of health problems that happens to babies whose mothers had a history of problem drinking during their pregnancy. There are a number of hazards:

• Babies may be smaller in weight and length.
• Despite good medical care, they may not catch up to normal babies.
• They may have small heads and may not grow well.
• They sometimes show abnormalities of the face.
• Most have some degree of learning and behavioural problems, such as attention deficit hyperactivity disorder or maladaptive behaviour, and learning difficulties.

FOR MORE INFORMATION ABOUT FASD CONTACT:

Canadian Centre on Substance Abuse:
1-613-235-4048
www.ccsa.ca

Motherisk Alcohol and Substance Use Helpline:
1–877–327–4636
www.motherisk.org

As children with FASD grow up, they tend to continue to have behavioural problems, learning problems in school, and trouble concentrating.

The rates of FASD in some segments of the population are much higher than the national average. Significant efforts have been developed to address FASD with these higher-risk groups with programs and initiatives that are respectful of culturally safe and culturally appropriate prevention, promotion and/or treatment. Visit Health Canada's website to get more information:

www.hc-sc.gc.ca/hl-vs/iyh-vsv/diseases-maladies/fasd-etcaf-eng.php

Street drugs

Using street drugs at any time during pregnancy may cause damage to your growing baby. Street drugs can be harmful to an adult, but babies are at much higher risk of harmful side effects. Babies born to mothers who use street drugs:

• may have brain damage that will affect their ability to learn,
• are usually smaller than other babies, and
• cry a lot and are more likely to be fussy.

If used often, some street drugs can even cause a baby to be born with an addiction.

If you are using street drugs, you need to stop before you get pregnant. If you do become pregnant while still using drugs, tell your health-care provider. Programs to help with quitting are available.

DO YOU HAVE AN ALCOHOL PROBLEM?

How many drinks does it take to make you feel the first effect (before pregnancy)?____(3 or more = 2 points)

Have your close friends or family worried or complained to you about your drinking in the past year? ____ (Yes = 2 points)

Do you sometimes take a drink in the morning when you first get up? ____ (Yes = 1 point)

Has a friend or family member ever told you about things you said or did while you were drinking that you could not remember?____ (Yes = 1 point)

Do you sometimes feel the need to reduce the amount you drink? ____ (Yes = 1 point)

Drinking any alcohol during pregnancy can harm your baby. If you scored 2 or more points, you may need extra help to stop drinking. Talk to your health-care provider.

Source: Russell M. New assessment tools for risk drinking during pregnancy: TWEAK. Alcohol Health and Research World 1994; 18 (1):55–61.

KEEPING TRACK OF MY PROGRESS

Date:

Blood pressure:

Weight:

THINGS TO DISCUSS WITH MY HEALTH-CARE PROVIDER:

☐ Concerns about my diet.

☐ The kind of work that I do.

☐ Quitting smoking.

☐ Concerns about alcohol or drugs.

☐ My medical history.

☐ My family history.

☐ Exercise.

Other concerns:

My pregnancy journal

My health before pregnancy

NUTRITION QUIZ:

I follow Canada's Food Guide.	Yes / No	I am taking folic acid.	Yes / No
I have enough calcium in my diet.	Yes / No	I have sources of vitamin C, vitamin D, magnesium, zinc, and omega-3 fatty acids in my diet.	Yes / No
I get enough iron from my diet.	Yes / No		

If you answer "No" to any of these questions (or are uncertain), review the chapter information, and talk to your health-care provider.

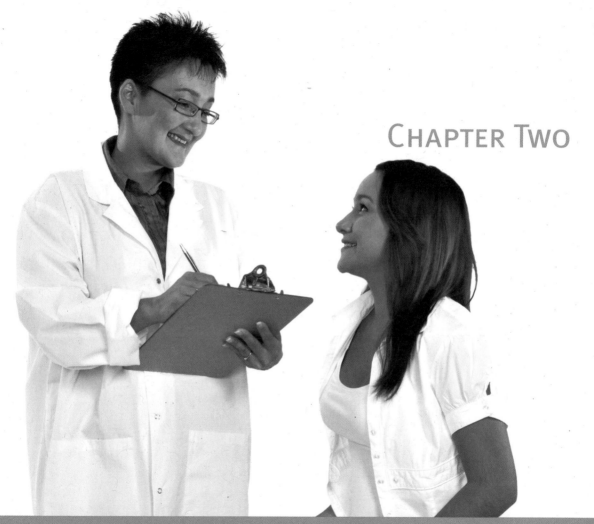

CHAPTER TWO

Off to a great start: the first trimester

It is common to divide the nine months of a full pregnancy into three **trimesters.** Each trimester is about three months long. The countdown begins at conception.

- The first trimester lasts for the 13 weeks after conception.

- The second trimester goes from the 13th week to about the 25th or 26th week.

- The third and final trimester lasts from about the 26th to the 40th week, when the baby is born.

Introduction

Your first trimester is the time when you and your baby will experience the greatest amount of change. During these 13 weeks, your baby will grow from a single cell to a little human being. At the same time, you will notice changes to your body that may surprise you, especially if this is your first pregnancy.

Finding out you are pregnant can be one of the most exciting moments of your life. This is especially true if you have been planning and hoping to become pregnant for some time. However, the first weeks of your pregnancy may bring some worry along with joy. What is happening to my body? What if something is wrong with my baby? Am I going to feel like this for nine months?

You will have lots of questions. Feeling some anxiety is perfectly normal. Your health-care team will have lots of tests that will provide answers. They will also be able to answer many of your direct questions and concerns.

To help you prepare, we'll explain the tests, as well as the main discomforts. Have you heard of morning sickness? We will talk about it. Sex? We will talk about it, too. Are you and your baby at risk from any kind of abuse? How can you get help? We will talk about this. What about prenatal classes, and exercise—especially Kegel exercises? Read on.

And, yes, because it does happen, we will discuss miscarriage. Your first trimester is when you are at greatest risk of having a miscarriage. Much of what we will cover in the next pages will help you to reduce those risks, but we will also address what happens if the worst happens.

Remember, by using this handbook and learning as much as you can about what will happen to you and your baby during pregnancy, you will be "off to a great start"! We are here to help you make choices about your health, diet, and lifestyle that will be best for you and your baby.

Your changing body

During your first trimester, your body will go through some dramatic changes. By the end of the first 13 weeks, you may not **look** very pregnant, but you will probably **feel** quite different.

At this stage, pregnancy hormones cause almost all the changes in your body. Remember *the placenta*? That's the small organ that grows along the inside wall of your uterus to nourish your baby. Well, it also produces hormones to help your body support your baby, too. This building process is complex and takes a lot of energy. That's why you feel so tired in your early months.

The changes in your body will not be very noticeable to other people. You may not even notice that your uterus is slowly growing—from the size of a pear to the size of a cantaloupe. Your milk glands develop and your breasts feel fuller, heavier, and more tender. Your heart works harder now because your body has produced extra blood to support the growing placenta and to provide oxygen and nutrients to your baby. You may be more aware of your breathing. Some women feel breathless because of hormone changes. The good news is that your menstrual cycle will stop. If you have any bleeding during pregnancy, consult your health-care provider right away.

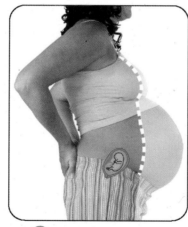

▶ *1ˢᵗ trimester*

Your growing baby

By the end of the first trimester, your 13-week old fetus will be about 9 cm long (3.5 inches) and weigh about 48 grams (1.7 ounces). Because the baby is so small, it will still have plenty of space to move around freely. Although it will be very active, you will not be able to feel the movement until later.

The baby's body will now be fully formed, but it will still need more time to gain weight and to allow its organs to mature. At 13 weeks, the fingers and toes are developed. The bones are mostly soft (cartilage), but they are starting to harden. The head still looks too big compared to the rest of the body. There are signs of 32 tooth buds in the jaw. The heart beats about 140 times per minute.

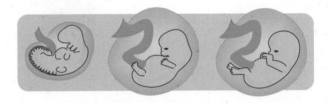

 The embryo develops rapidly during the first eight weeks of pregnancy.

How often should I expect to visit my health-care provider?

Your first visit will include lots of testing—head to toe. For the rest of the first trimester, you should see your health-care provider at least once every four weeks. After 30 weeks, the visits are usually increased to once every two to three weeks. After 36 weeks, you should see your health-care provider every week or two until you go into labour.

Your first prenatal visit

You should book your first prenatal visit as soon as you learn you are pregnant. Be prepared, because this visit is more in-depth and longer than the rest. Some doctors call it a "head-to-toe." Expect to have a complete check-up. It may even include a pregnancy test to confirm your pregnancy and an internal physical exam of your reproductive organs and pelvis.

You will be asked to provide details about your medical history and other births and pregnancies. You will be asked if your immunizations are up-to-date. If you saw your health-care provider when you were planning to get pregnant, you may discuss some of the same topics you discussed then. During this visit, your health-care provider will also calculate your due date. Again, this is done by counting from the first day of your last menstrual period. That's why it's important that you know this date for your first visit.

Your health-care provider knows how important it is for you to be well-informed about your pregnancy and your developing baby. This visit is also a good time to have a discussion about how to prepare for breastfeeding. But office visits, even this first long one, may not cover every topic. That's why you should read educational materials such as this handbook and attend prenatal classes.

About weight gain

Weight gain during pregnancy is necessary. It supports the growth of the fetus and the placenta, as well as changes in your body, such as an increased volume of blood and fluid, larger breast size, and some storage of fat.

The amount of weight gain that is right for you depends on your BMI before you got pregnant. BMI stands for "body mass index." It is an excellent way to estimate the best weight for a person's height. Your

WHAT IS MY DUE DATE?

The Big Day—your due date—is calculated by counting nine calendar months, plus seven days from the first day of your last menstrual period. Now you know why it's important to keep track of the dates of your monthly cycle! (Tell your friends.)

About 85% of babies are born within a week of (before or after) their due date.

Pregnant women may not need to increase their caloric intake during the first trimester, but should eat to satisfy their appetite—ideally, three meals and three snacks, spread throughout the day. A healthy snack includes at least two of the four food groups (such as half a sandwich—try turkey-and-tomato, made with whole grain bread—and a glass of milk).

By the last trimester, even if you feel less hungry because your growing baby is putting pressure on your stomach, you still have increased needs. You should continue eating healthy foods, and don't forget the three meals and three snacks.

health-care provider can calculate your BMI based on your height and weight and let you know if you are overweight, underweight, or at the ideal weight. You can also calculate your BMI using this formula: BMI = weight(kg)/height(m)^2. The BMI monogram is not intended for use for those under 18 years of age, or for pregnant or lactating women.

Health Risk Classification According to Body Mass Index (BMI)*		
Classification	BMI Category (kg/m²)	Risk of developing health problems
Underweight	Less than 18.5	Increased
Normal Weight	18.5–24.9	Least
Overweight	25.0–29.9	Increased
Obese class I	30.0–34.9	High
Obese class II	35.0–39.9	Very high
Obese class III	More than or equal to 40.0	Extremely high

*Source: Canadian guidelines for Body Weight Classification in Adults, Health Canada. Reproduced with the permission of the Minister of Public Works and Government Services Canada, 2008.

The correct amount of weight to gain during pregnancy is based on your own weight profile. The table (see page 41) provides guidelines, but it may not accurately reflect the risk of gaining *too much weight*. Recent studies show a link between high average and excessive weight gain in pregnant women and the likelihood of children born from those pregnancies to become overweight by age five. Women who gain too much weight are also shown to have a greater risk of poor infant outcomes, including oversized babies. On the other hand, not gaining enough weight during pregnancy can also be a problem. This applies especially to young adolescent women (teenagers) who still have their own growing to do.

Weight Gain During Pregnancy*	
BMI before pregnancy	Recommended Weight Gain
BMI less than 19.8	12.5 to 18 kg (28 to 40 lb)
BMI between 19.8 to 26	11.5 to 16 kg (25 to 35 lb)
BMI between 26 to 29	7 to 11.5 kg (15 to 25 lb)
BMI more than 29	at least 6 kg (15 lb)
Twin pregnancies	16 to 20.5 kg (35 to 45 lb)
Other	Young women (teenagers) should strive for gains at the upper end of the ranges. Short women (less than 157 cm) should aim for gains at the lower end of their range.

* Reprinted with permission from Table 1.1, "Nutrition During Pregnancy: Part I: Weight Gain, Part II: Nutrient Supplements"© 1990 by the National Academy of Sciences, Courtesy of the National Academies Press, Washington, D.C.

Recommended weight gain is subject to change. To get the most up-to-date information on weight gain during pregnancy, visit the Institute of Medicine website at www.iom.edu.

For more details about nutrition and pregnancy, see Chapter One.

About vitamin supplements

Prenatal vitamins contain many of the extra nutrients you need during pregnancy, such as folic acid and iron. (See Chapter One for more details on vitamins.) If your diet excludes foods from an entire food group, you may need other supplements. But talk to your health-care provider first. The best source of the nutrients you need can be found in a healthy diet.

ARE YOU SOMEONE WHO NEEDS MORE CALORIES?

☐ I am having twins or multiples.

☐ I am a teenager.

☐ I am very physically active.

☐ I have had a baby with low birth weight (baby weighed less than 5.5 pounds at birth).

☐ I am thin (underweight).

☐ I am going through a lot of emotional stress.

If you checked off any of the boxes above, speak to your health-care provider. You might need more calories during pregnancy.

Be aware of your special need for iron, folic acid, and essential fatty acids.

Refer to the nutrition section in Chapter One.

WHY DO I NEED TO SEE MY HEALTH-CARE PROVIDER WHEN I FEEL FINE?

Prenatal care is the term for the medical care you receive before your baby is born. Almost 90% of pregnancies and babies are "normal," and studies show that women who have regular prenatal care have better pregnancies and healthy babies. To help you ensure you are part of the "normal" segment, you should make an appointment as soon as you know you are pregnant. Set up your appointments in advance—especially if you live in a remote area (see page 45, Getting to appointments).

Also, getting to know your health-care provider—especially at an early stage—will make it more comfortable for you to share your concerns and ask your questions openly. Regular check-ups also make it easier for your health-care provider to spot any possible problems early on so you can take steps to try to prevent any harm from coming to you or your baby.

"GOING IT ALONE"

Perhaps you are pregnant and don't have a partner for support. Other people can help, including your family and friends. Find people you can trust and talk with.

- *Make a list of the things you need help with. Ask friends and family to help you.*

- *Early on, ask someone you trust to be your birth partner. You can always change your mind later.*

- *Take someone with you to your health-care provider appointments, scans, or tests.*

- *Go shopping with friends or family to buy the things you need for the baby . . . and for yourself!*

If you are a teenager, talk to a health-care provider or other community resource person about the support your community may offer.

Discussing your pregnancy

You will want to be able to talk honestly with your health-care team during your pregnancy. They will have some important questions and you should think about how you will answer them ahead of time.

- Tell them how you feel about the pregnancy.
- Talk about your partner and the role he or she may play during the pregnancy.
- Tell them if you feel safe or unsafe, loved or not loved, and about the kind of bond you have with your partner.

- Explain how your family and friends feel about this pregnancy.
- Find out where you can go for prenatal classes and what you can do to keep you and your baby as healthy as possible.

Remember to take this journal with you each time you see your health-care provider. We have left space at the end of the chapter so you can write down questions for your health-care provider, as well as the answers.

You are expecting twins . . . or more!

If you know you will be giving birth to twins, triplets, or more, you are not alone! In Canada, 3% of births are multiples, and that number is rising. You might be feeling excited and overwhelmed at the same time. How will you cope? What kind of care will you and your babies need? There will be many joys, but what are the risks?

The fact that you are expecting multiples means that you will need special health care and support while you are pregnant. The biggest risk is having a preterm birth (see page 77).

The good news is that because multiple births are more common, the health-care systems are well-equipped to deal with them. Early and regular health care and support will be important in helping you avoid problems with your pregnancy and birth. Your health-care provider will likely recommend that you have appointments with a specialist (such as an obstetrician or a doctor who specializes in multiple births).

LIST OF REGISTRATION AND
CONTACT INFORMATION, DATES,
LOCATIONS, AND TIMES FOR
PRENATAL CLASSES

You can get more details about multiple births from:

- The Society of Obstetricians and Gynaecologists of Canada's Consensus Statement on the Management of Twin Pregnancies at www.sogc.org.
- Multiple Births Canada's website at www.multiplebirthscanada.org
- The Toronto Centre for Multiple Births at Sunnybrook Hospital in Toronto, 1-416-323-6340

Prenatal classes

Thousands of women and their families take part in prenatal classes every year. Classes are very helpful for women who are having their first baby and for young women who are pregnant during their teen years. Learning about pregnancy also helps women to make informed decisions about their pregnancy and about childbirth. Women say they feel more confident when they understand the changes that pregnancy brings.

At one time, prenatal classes focused only on the stages of labour and on pain control during delivery. Today's classes still deal with these topics, but they also explore other vital topics such as breastfeeding, prenatal nutrition, parenting skills, signs of problems, and exercise during pregnancy.

Prenatal classes also include partners, support people, and sometimes even children. When partners go to classes, they can learn about their changing relationship and their new role as parents. Children can learn to prepare for the birth of a new brother or sister.

Some prenatal classes are designed to respect different ethnic or cultural backgrounds. They may be offered in languages other than English or French. Other classes focus on the needs of teens or are tailored to the specific needs of Aboriginal communities. Some prenatal classes help families adjust to their new baby by exploring topics such as breastfeeding, getting back into shape, sex after pregnancy, and normal infant growth.

If you would like to be part of prenatal or postnatal classes, ask your health-care provider about what exists in your community and how you can register for classes.

Travel during pregnancy

Travel is easiest before your 20th week of pregnancy. After 20 weeks, whether you travel should depend on:

- where you plan to travel
- how you will travel
- the distance you will travel
- the length of time you will be away from home (and your health-care provider)

A quick flight will be different from a long car ride across the country, or a trip overseas. Before you plan a trip, you should always talk to your health-care provider. Then, you should carry all the basic details about your pregnancy with you. This includes your blood type and the results of your latest ultrasound. This information may help you in case of an emergency or if you are faced with something you did not plan.

Sex during pregnancy

When they are pregnant, many women feel a change in their levels of sexual desire.

In most cases, having intercourse will not harm the pregnancy in any way. However, your health-care provider may tell you to avoid or limit intercourse if you have:

GETTING TO APPOINTMENTS

In some provinces and territories, if you live in a remote area and must travel far away to an urban centre for special medical care, you may be able to apply for and receive a government travel grant. Ask your health-care provider if this applies to you.

Some First Nations, Métis and Inuit people may have access to Health Canada's Non-Insured Health Benefits Program to help pay for medical transportation and other health-care costs during pregnancy and childbirth. To learn more about this program, contact your Non-Insured Health Benefits Regional Office or visit their website at www.hc-sc.gc.ca.

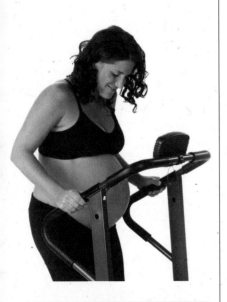

- an infection
- bleeding
- problems with leaking amniotic fluid
- the breaking of the amniotic sac

Based on your circumstances, you should continue to use condoms to protect you and your growing baby from sexually transmitted infections.

Some couples feel closer during this special time and continue to enjoy sex until just before their baby is due. Other couples feel their relationship is strained by all the changes taking place. They find that sex is not as fulfilling during pregnancy. Your partner may be worried that having sex could harm the baby. If either of you is uncomfortable about sexual relations, make time for other kinds of physical touch. You can cuddle with each other, hold hands, give or get a massage, or take a bath together.

If you are comfortable with the idea, you can explore alternatives to vaginal sex such as masturbation and oral sex. Just a warning about oral sex: ask your partner to be very careful **not to blow any air into your vagina**. Doing this could force air into your bloodstream, which could be fatal to both you and your baby.

Exercise during pregnancy

Whether you are pregnant or not, exercise is good for you. However, it's important that you not overdo the exercise program you choose. We suggest you try different workouts that can be part of your daily routine: aerobic exercise (with caution), strength training, yoga, and tai chi.

Aerobic exercise

Exercise that makes your heart beat faster than when you are resting is called aerobic exercise. It can include brisk walking, jogging, riding a bike, swimming, or team sports.

If you have been active before you became pregnant, you can likely continue with the same, or a slightly lower, level of activity. Discuss your exercise plans with your health-care provider early in your pregnancy to make sure you do not have any health problems that would make vigorous exercise risky. Most women who are runners can continue to run when they are pregnant without harming their growing baby. If you feel pain in the pubic region, this is a sign that your body is not adapting well to running and you should stop.

Exercise is good for both the mother and the baby and you can begin to exercise during your second trimester without fear of miscarriage or labour problems. If you haven't been physically active at least two to three times per week before becoming pregnant, you should wait until your second trimester to begin exercising, and only do so after you discuss your choices with your health-care provider.

If you are worried about exercising too hard, try the "talk test." It's very simple: you should always be able to carry on a conversation during your workout. Otherwise, reduce your level of effort.

Once your health-care provider says it's okay to exercise, begin to do so. Walk, swim, or join a fitness class. Some classes are designed just for pregnant women and new mothers. If you are part of a regular aerobics class, talk to your teacher about what you might need to avoid (routines that are high-impact or that put stress on your lower back).

Strength training

Building and maintaining muscle mass is an important part of any exercise program. But be cautious! Remember to breathe continuously and smoothly during each part of the weight training movement. Talk to your health-care provider before you begin or continue a weight-training program.

WHEN IS IT NOT SAFE TO EXERCISE?

As you read this list, check off any of the statements that are true for you.

☐ *I have heart problems.*

☐ *I have a serious lung condition and/or breathing problems.*

☐ *I have high blood pressure.*

☐ *I have experienced bleeding from my vagina during this pregnancy.*

☐ *I have low levels of iron in my blood (anemia).*

☐ *I am carrying more than one baby.*

☐ *I have problems controlling my blood sugar levels.*

☐ *I have concerns about my blood sugar levels.*

☐ *My health-care provider has told me the fetus is too small for its age.*

☐ *I am at high risk for preterm labour.*

☐ *I am very underweight or have been diagnosed with an eating disorder.*

☐ *I suspect I have a rupture of the membranes.*

If you have ticked any of the boxes above, you should not exercise during your pregnancy until you have discussed your condition with your health-care provider.

AM I EXERCISING TOO HARD?

As you read this list, check off any of the statements that are true for you.

☐ I feel exhausted during my workout.

☐ I feel very hot and dehydrated when I exercise.

☐ I have trouble talking when I exercise.

☐ I have chest pain, jaw pain, or unexplained arm pain.

☐ I feel dizzy during or after exercise.

If you ticked any of the boxes above, you are overexerting yourself during your workout. It would be best to reduce the level of your exercise routine and talk to your health-care provider.

THE TALK TEST

You should always be able to carry on a conversation when you are exercising. If you cannot, you are working too hard. If you can, you are doing great.

For more advice on exercise during pregnancy, call the Exercise and Pregnancy Helpline at 1-866-93-SPORT (77678). It is a service provided by Physicians, Physiotherapists, and Athletic Therapists at Sport C.A.R.E., Women's College Hospital, and is affiliated with Motherisk at the Hospital for Sick Children. The helpline is a voicemail system that allows you to ask any questions you may have about exercise during pregnancy. Within 24 hours, a sports medicine physician or trained athletic therapist will return your call. These professionals can help you decide on the kind of exercises that are safe for you and provide you with educational materials.

Rules to follow when you exercise

Aerobic exercise

This kind of exercise uses the large muscle groups. It includes walking, running, swimming, stationary bikes, low-impact aerobics, cross-country skiing, and aquafit.

- During pregnancy, you should limit your aerobic exercise sessions to 30 to 40 minutes, including the warm-up and cool-down. Warm-up is a time for your body to adjust to an increase in heart rate and circulation. It is best to begin your activity slowly, at low intensity, and to gradually increase your movement for 5 to 8 minutes. For runners, this means your first 5 to 8 minutes should be variable speed walking to increase your pace. Cool-down will take another 5 to 8 minutes and should consist of slowing your body down by doing some deep breathing and slow stretching.
- Take rest breaks when you feel you need them. Keep your heart rate at the low end of the target heart rate for women your age. Check yourself by using the "talk test."
- You should drink one glass of water every exercise session. You can drink it 30 minutes before or right after the session. The important thing is to keep well hydrated every day and not just when you are exercising.

- Be careful when you are doing sports that require balance and co-ordination. During your pregnancy, your centre of gravity will be constantly changing.
- Avoid contact sports and any activity that might make you fall or be hit. This includes downhill skiing, mountain climbing, floor hockey, water skiing, and soccer.

Strength training

Avoid any exercise that causes you to hold your breath and bear down at the same time, such as heavy weight-lifting routines.

After the fourth month of pregnancy, you should change your abdominal exercises. Stop lying on your back when you do them. Instead, lie on your side or do the exercise while you are standing.

You should avoid stretching ligaments and tendons too much. This becomes more likely because they may be more flexible due to pregnancy hormones. Yoga and Pilates have not been studied in pregnancy. If qualified intructors know you are pregnant, they will suggest ways for you to adjust the poses so you can be safe.

The most important muscles to tone when you are pregnant are the pelvic muscles. (See page 50 to learn about Kegel exercises.) They help develop pelvic and core strength. Core stability takes some stress off the pelvic floor and prevents your body from using your pelvic muscles too much.

At the gym or fitness centre

Avoid exercises that strain your lower back. Always maintain good posture.

Also, be careful of your body temperature, especially if exercising in warm and humid environments (either indoors or outdoors). Always be aware of increasing your body heat—which could happen in hot tubs,

---

EXERCISE SAFETY CONSIDERATIONS

- *Avoid exercise in warm/humid environments, especially during the first trimester.*

- *Avoid isometric exercise or straining while you are holding your breath.*

- *Maintain adequate nutrition and hydration. Drink liquids before and after exercise.*

- *Avoid exercising while lying on your back past the fourth month of pregnancy.*

- *Avoid activities that involve physical contact or danger of falling.*

- *Know your limits. Pregnancy is not a good time to train for an athletic competition.*

- *Know the reasons to stop exercise and consult a qualified health-care provider immediately if they occur.*

Source: Physical Activity Readiness Medical Examination for pregnancy (PARmed-X for Pregnancy) © 2002. Used with permission from the Canadian Society for Exercise Physiology www.csep.ca. If you have Internet access, you can download the complete guideline questionnaire from: http://uwfitness.uwaterloo .ca/PDF/parmed-xpreg_000.pdf.

PELVIC TILTS MAY HELP TO RELIEVE YOUR BACKACHE

Do this simple exercise two or three times a day. It will strengthen your abdominal muscles and take some pressure off your aching back.

- *Lie on the floor and relax your back.*

- *Exhale and pull your buttocks forward, pulling your pubic bone upward while keeping your lower back on the floor.*

- *Hold this position for a count of three, then inhale and relax.*

- *Repeat five times.*

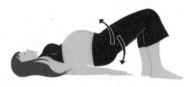

 Pelvic tilt

saunas, and steam rooms. Your baby's body temperature may rise and that is something you must avoid. Warm weather exercise should be balanced by drinking lots of fluids.

Kegel exercises strengthen your core and pelvic floor muscles

Kegel exercises provide strength training for the muscles that surround your pelvic floor. Kegel exercises will also help prevent a flow of urine when you cough, lift, or laugh. By learning this routine, you will develop a good habit for life. It helps you get back in shape after childbirth. It will also help you prevent urine flow problems (also called urinary stress incontinence) later in life.

1. Relax and sit or stand comfortably.

2. Find your pelvic muscle. Imagine that you are trying to hold back urine, or a bowel movement. Squeeze the muscles you would use to do that.

3. Tighten the muscles for 5 to 10 seconds.

4. Do not hold your breath—breathe normally.

5. Do not tighten your stomach or buttocks—keep them relaxed.

6. Now relax the muscles for about 10 seconds.

7. Repeat the squeeze–hold–relax routine, 12 to 20 times.

Why do I need to have so many tests?

When you go to your first prenatal visit, your health-care provider will recommend a number of routine laboratory tests. These help to find or predict risks to your health and the health of your baby. They may include:

Blood tests

How many tests you will have depends on your medical history. Here is the complete list:

- **Blood type and antibodies**: to identify your blood group and rhesus (Rh) factor. This test also looks for any unusual antibodies in your blood. (See page 56, Blood types and Rh factors.)
- **Hemoglobin**: to check your blood to make sure it can carry enough iron and oxygen. (See page 28, What is anemia?)
- **Hepatitis B surface antigens:** to see if you have been exposed to hepatitis B. (See page 58, Hepatitis B.)
- **HIV:** to check whether you have been exposed to HIV, the virus that causes AIDS. (See page 59, HIV and AIDS.)
- **Rubella titre:** to see if you have immunity to rubella (German measles). (See page 57, Rubella (German measles) or varicella (chicken pox).)
- **Varicella (chicken pox):** to see if you have immunity to this virus. If you had chicken pox when you were younger, your body will have immunity and you will not need to have this test. (See page 57, Rubella (German measles) or varicella (chicken pox).)
- **Syphilis screening:** to see if you have been exposed to syphilis, a sexually transmitted infection.

Pap test: to check for cancer of the cervix or abnormal cells that could lead to cancer.

Urine test: to check sugar and protein levels in your urine, and to make sure you do not have a urinary tract infection. This kind of infection can be treated. But without treatment, your risk of preterm labour rises.

Remember the talk about your medical history at the start of your pregnancy? Well, you should also find out about your family's medical history, as well as the medical history of the birth father's family—before your 9th week. You should let your health-care provider know if either family has any of the following conditions:

☐ *Congenital heart defect*

☐ *Spina bifida*

☐ *Anencephaly*

☐ *Cleft palate*

☐ *Clubfoot*

☐ *Huntington's disease*

☐ *Born with extra fingers or toes*

☐ *Sickle cell disease*

☐ *Tay-Sachs disease*

☐ *Cystic fibrosis*

☐ *Thalassemia*

☐ *Hemophilia*

☐ *Muscular dystrophy*

☐ *Fragile x syndrome*

☐ *Down syndrome*

☐ *Other* _____

Genetic screening

When a health problem is **hereditary,** this means it is passed through the genes of the mother or the father to a child, the same way as eye colour or hair colour. Sometimes, these kinds of health problems can be found using special tests that will require a referral to a genetic specialist.

At your first prenatal visit, your health-care provider will talk about:

• blood-screening tests for certain genetic disorders
• ultrasound

Almost 90% of pregnancies in Canada result in the birth of a healthy baby. However, if there are any problems or risks, knowing about them before the baby is born can help families and health-care providers plan for the future and for any special medical care or treatment that might be needed.

In Canada, genetic screening is offered to all women. The type of testing that you get depends on what screening programs are available in your area.

Testing may be done using blood tests and ultrasound, or both combined. Other tests may be needed if it seems you are at higher risk of giving birth to a child with certain types of conditions or medical problems.

Tests are important. Some tests are "routine"—used during all pregnancies. Others are used only when certain details are needed to identify a condition. Many of them are expensive. Using all tests during all pregnancies would quickly overload our health-care system.

Your health-care provider will also tell you that no test is 100% accurate and no single test covers all possible conditions. You need to know that there are risks, as well as benefits, to testing. For example, some tests need a tissue or fluid sample from the baby. This may involve inserting a needle into your abdomen to take the sample. Doing this is common, but there is a small risk. Your health-care provider will discuss the need for certain tests, any risks involved, and then he or she will make a recommendation. In the end, you will be the one who decides whether to have a test or not.

Tests that check your baby's health before it is born

There are many types of tests that can check your baby's development. Some are offered to all women early on and throughout the pregnancy (such as ultrasound). Other tests, like amniocentesis, are only offered if there is a specific concern or possible risk. Some tests can pose a small risk to the mother and/or the baby and some cost a lot of money. Do not expect your health-care provider to give you a test unless you need it.

Ultrasound

Most people have heard about ultrasound. What they need to know is that it should only be done for medical reasons—not for commercial gain or entertainment. One of the purposes of ultrasound is to confirm your baby's due date. It is recommended that you have an ultrasound test at least once, usually at 18 weeks of pregnancy.

The test uses sound waves to create a picture of your baby on a computer screen. You, your family, and your health-care providers will be able to see a real-time, shaded image of the baby. Ultrasound is also used for these reasons:

- to see the baby's position
- to check the baby's growth and well-being
- to find out where the placenta is attached to the uterus
- to see if there is more than one baby
- to check for some abnormalities

ULTRASOUND

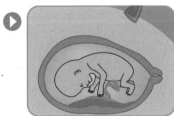

ULTRASOUND

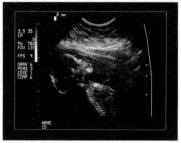

An ultrasound takes pictures by converting sound waves that can travel safely into your body. The ultrasound technician will apply gel to your belly. This gel helps a small hand-held device called a transducer (which sends the sound waves that connect to the screen that shows your baby) to move easily over your skin. You might feel light pressure on your belly, but you will not feel any pain. Most ultrasound exams last about 30 minutes. If your health-care provider has asked for more details from an ultrasound, the test could take longer.

Before you go for an ultrasound, you will learn how to prepare and where to go for the test. Sometimes, you will be told to arrive with a full bladder. This helps the sound waves travel through the skin and tissues to get a better picture of your baby.

Some women might need to have the ultrasound done through the vagina. The ultrasound technician uses a special transducer that is inserted into the vagina. This should not hurt.

Maternal serum screening (MSS)

You may have heard of MSS—a blood test that measures substances in the mother's blood called "markers." High levels of these markers may show that the baby is at risk for certain conditions. Positive results only indicate a higher risk. Other tests will need to be done to confirm this. If MSS is offered in your area, your health-care provider will give you reading material to help you decide whether or not to have this testing done.

Nuchal translucency

This special type of ultrasound is offered in some areas to screen for Down syndrome. The test is given between the 11th and 14th week of pregnancy. It measures the thickness of the layer of fluid at the back of the baby's neck. If the layer is thicker than average, this means a higher likelihood of Down syndrome. A woman will then be offered a test called amniocentesis (see below). Both amniocentesis and MSS may be used to make a more accurate diagnosis regarding certain genetic disorders.

Chorionic villus sampling (CVS)

This is another test for genetic-related disorders. It is done between the 10th and 12th weeks of pregnancy. The doctor uses an ultrasound to pass a small needle through the cervix or the abdomen, into the placenta, to take a sample of special cells (chorionic villi).

Amniocentesis

A number of genetic or inherited disorders can be identified by taking a sample of the amniotic fluid that surrounds the baby. This test is done after the 14th week of pregnancy. A fine needle is inserted into the uterus via the abdomen. Ultrasound helps the doctor find a safe place to insert the needle. It may take up to four weeks to get the full results of this test.

Fetal tissue and blood sampling

Other tests allow doctors to take samples of fetal tissue (from the skin, the liver, the abdomen, or other organs). As with amniocentesis, the doctor uses an ultrasound to guide a small needle into the target area on the unborn baby's body or umbilical cord (for a blood sample).

CHORIONIC VILLUS SAMPLING

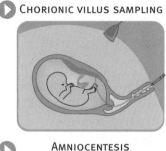

AMNIOCENTESIS

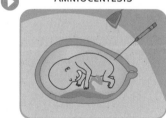

Blood types and Rh factors

When you are pregnant, you will need to know your blood type. This will be done during your first series of tests. Why? Although it is not likely that you will need a blood transfusion during your pregnancy or during the birth, if you do, the health-care providers need to know what type of blood to give you. There are four blood types: O, A, B, and AB. Type O blood is the most common type in North America.

You may have also heard of "Rh factor" in people's blood. Everyone's blood is either Rh positive or Rh negative.

A baby's blood type and Rh factor depend on their parents' blood types and Rh factors—just like eye colour, skin colour, or hair colour. A baby may have the blood type and the Rh factor of either parent, or a combination of both parents' types and factors.

Only 15% of the population is Rh negative. Problems may occur if the mother is Rh negative and the baby is Rh positive. At one time, this blood incompatibility could lead to Rh disease and could even cause the death of the baby. Now, health-care providers know how to prevent Rh disease and it has become very rare. If your blood test shows you might be at risk of passing along Rh disease, you will get Rh-immune globulin (RhIg) between the 28th and 32nd weeks of pregnancy and again after your baby's birth, or at any time during pregnancy if bleeding occurs.

Fifth disease

Fifth disease is a common viral illness among children. It is caused by parvovirus B19. It is usually very mild and appears in children as a red rash on the face, trunk, arms and legs. If you are pregnant and you often spend time with young children, you may come in contact with the disease. However, more than half of women have been infected once and are now immune. Women who get the infection may have fever, a rash, and joint pain. Most women have no symptoms and no serious complications. In very rare cases, the virus can infect an unborn baby and cause illness or death.

If a pregnant woman is exposed to, or shows signs of, a parvovirus infection, she should have her blood tested to see if she is already immune. Certain women are at a higher risk of being exposed to this. They include daycare workers, schoolteachers, and mothers of young children. However, there is no proof that women reduce their risk of infection by leaving work. If you spend a lot of time with children, washing your hands frequently helps to decrease your chance of infection. If you are pregnant and think you may have been exposed to this virus, talk to your health-care provider.

Rubella (German measles) or varicella (chicken pox)

Both rubella and varicella can cause serious problems for a growing baby. That's why it is best to make sure that you are immune before you get pregnant. If you are vaccinated before becoming pregnant, wait at least one month before you try to conceive.

If you are not immune to either rubella or varicella and you are pregnant, your health-care provider will discuss the risks and options with you. Pregnant women should avoid being immunized against rubella or varicella; however, you may be vaccinated after giving birth.

Hepatitis B

There are several types of hepatitis, a viral infection that affects the liver. Hepatitis B is the type that can affect babies during pregnancy. It can be spread during sexual contact, or passed to a baby during childbirth. It is the most serious type of hepatitis to have during pregnancy. One in every 250 people has this disease. It is more common in people who have recently moved to Canada from Asia.

Many people with hepatitis B have no symptoms and do not even know they have it. They are called chronic carriers and they can pass hepatitis B on to other people. A small percentage of chronic carriers will develop very serious liver disease that can cause death.

Without treatment, about 50% of babies born to mothers who test positive for hepatitis B will be infected. This usually happens during birth or while breastfeeding. Without treatment, many of these babies will become chronic carriers and a few may develop long-term health problems.

The good news is that babies born to mothers who test positive for hepatitis B can be treated soon after birth. They will receive both the hepatitis B immune globulin and the hepatitis B vaccine. With treatment, 95% of these babies will not be infected, nor will they become carriers.

Herpes

Herpes is a virus that causes cold sores and genital infections. At least 10% of people have one of the two forms called Herpes Simplex Virus (HSV). While the virus is not life-threatening to adults, it can spread easily between sexual partners and can be painful and troublesome. Pregnant women should know about herpes because the virus can infect your baby during delivery and cause serious harm.

The most common type of herpes infection is HSV-1, the type that causes cold sores on the face, mostly on the lips. The other, HSV-2, occurs on the

Am I at risk for hepatitis B?

☐ I have had a blood transfusion or blood products for a clotting disorder.

☐ I have had more than one sexual partner.

☐ I have injected drugs.

☐ I have shared needles when I injected drugs.

☐ I have handled blood or blood products at my job.

☐ I was born in Asia.

If you checked one or more boxes, you are at higher risk of having hepatitis B.

If you have hepatitis B, a vaccine can protect your baby.

sex organs (genitals) of both men and women. But either type of herpes can infect the face or genitals.

What are the risks of herpes to your baby?

The greatest danger to your baby comes during delivery. The baby may get neonatal herpes if you already have herpes. While this is rare, it is also life-threatening and can create skin, eye, and mouth infections, and damage to the baby's central nervous system and other internal organs.

What should you do if you or your partner has herpes?

You should tell your health-care provider if you suspect that you or your partner have either type of herpes. You should avoid sexual intercourse and oral sex with partners who have, or you suspect may have, an active herpes outbreak.

Having a genital herpes infection for the first time, near the time of delivery, is the greatest risk to your baby. If you have genital herpes, your health-care provider may suggest you take anti-viral medications during the last four weeks of pregnancy. This will decrease the chance of an outbreak at delivery. If you have an outbreak at the time of delivery, then a Caesarean section will probably be recommended.

HIV and AIDS

Human Immunodeficiency Virus (HIV) is found in an infected person's body fluids. This includes semen, blood, vaginal fluids, and breast milk. HIV causes infections and diseases that harm a person's immune and nervous systems. HIV can lead to Acquired Immune Deficiency Syndrome (AIDS)—the name of the disease caused by HIV that can lead to death.

Symptoms of HIV may take five years or more to appear. Many people with HIV do not know they have it. But HIV can be found in a simple blood test. The most common way for the virus to spread from an

---

DO I HAVE A LIFESTYLE THAT PUTS ME AT RISK FOR SEXUALLY TRANSMITTED INFECTIONS (STIs)?

☐ *I have had many sexual partners.*

☐ *I have had sex with many partners, some of whom did not wear a condom.*

☐ *I use street drugs.*

☐ *I inject street drugs.*

☐ *I have a drinking problem.*

☐ *I participate in anal sex.*

If you agree with any of these statements, you are at higher risk of having a sexually transmitted infection. You should be tested for STIs (including AIDS).

infected person to a non-infected person is during sex. However, the virus can also enter a person's bloodstream through a needle that carries the virus. You will be at risk if you share needles with an HIV-positive intravenous drug user. It is very rare to get an HIV infection from a blood transfusion. In Canada, this is no longer a high risk because the blood supply is now carefully screened for HIV.

You can reduce your chances of getting HIV by:

• asking questions about your partner's sexual past before you have sexual contact
• limiting the number of sexual partners you have

Ideally, when you begin a new relationship, you should use a condom for at least six months. After two negative HIV tests by both people, it is probably safe to stop using condoms—as long as you have also been tested for other sexually transmitted infections and neither of you has had other sexual partners. If you use injection drugs, never share needles.

The number of women of childbearing age who are infected with HIV is rising. A pregnant woman can pass the virus on to her child during pregnancy, childbirth, or while breastfeeding. Women who know they are HIV positive can greatly reduce their baby's chance of getting the virus (down to 1%) if they receive treatment throughout pregnancy and during labour, and if the baby gets treatment during the first six weeks of life.

That is why every woman who is pregnant, or thinking about getting pregnant, should be tested for HIV. The choice is yours. All pregnant women in Canada are offered HIV testing during pregnancy.

Diabetes

Some women develop diabetes during pregnancy; this is called **gestational diabetes** and is discussed in Chapter Three. Diabetes is a disease in which the body does not produce or properly use insulin.

The two most common types of diabetes, Type 1 and Type 2, affect both women and men. Diabetes happens when a person's body (and more specifically the pancreas) does not produce enough insulin. Insulin is a hormone that tells the cells how to convert sugars and starches into energy. Without this form of energy . . . well, life cannot exist.

Types of Diabetes	
Type 1	Type 2
When the pancreas fails to produce any insulin at all.	When the pancreas fails to produce enough insulin or when the body cannot use this insulin properly.
↓	↓
A person with Type 1 diabetes must inject insulin to allow glucose (sugars from food) to enter and fuel the cells of the body.	A person with Type 2 diabetes may be able to control their blood sugars (glucose levels) by eating properly and by getting enough regular exercise to burn off extra glucose.

If you have Type 1 (insulin-dependent) diabetes

People with Type 1 diabetes must test their blood glucose levels every day and then inject the right amount of insulin to keep those levels normal. For some people, having good control of their blood glucose levels is not easy. When a woman who must use insulin becomes pregnant, this challenge becomes even greater.

Good control of blood glucose levels is very important for a healthy pregnancy, especially during the month when the baby is conceived and during the first trimester. Babies born to mothers whose blood glucose levels are not under tight control during their entire pregnancy may be unusually large (4.5 kg/10 lbs or more) and hard to deliver, or they may have birth defects. During your pregnancy, eating a healthy balanced diet that includes three meals and three snacks a day, avoiding sugar, and exercising will help your own and your baby's health.

DENTAL HEALTH IS
IMPORTANT IN PREGNANCY

Do you have problems with your teeth or jaw?

Do you brush and floss your teeth regularly?

When was the last time you saw your dentist?

If you have tooth decay, sore or bleeding gums, or have not seen your dentist in the last 6 to 12 months, make a dental appointment. It is both safe and important to visit a dentist during your pregnancy.

A woman with diabetes should be monitored by a health-care team. This team should include someone who is a diabetes expert. As her pregnancy advances, the team must make sure her blood sugar level is well controlled.

About dental health

The hormonal changes that come with pregnancy can also affect your teeth and gums. Some women notice that their gums become swollen or may even bleed. It's an important time to keep any regular dental appointments and to brush and floss regularly. New research reveals that pregnant women with tooth decay and gum disease are at higher risk for preterm delivery. Talk to your dentist if you have questions or problems. If you do not have access to a dentist, please see your community health nurse.

Common discomforts in early pregnancy

Nausea and vomiting

We still do not know what causes "morning sickness." It happens most often during the first three or four months of pregnancy, but sometimes it can last longer. You may feel nauseated at any time during the day or night and when your stomach is empty.

For most women, the feeling of nausea and the number of times they vomit will ease up a bit at some point during the day. This gives them a chance to feel hungry again and to eat food that will stay in their stomachs. However, 1% of pregnant women in Canada (about 4,000 women per year) will suffer from such severe nausea and vomiting that the lack of food, fluids, and nutrients may be harmful to their health and the well-being of their baby.

If it is not treated, severe nausea and vomiting can cause a woman to lose weight and can create an electrolyte imbalance. Electrolytes—such as sodium, calcium, chloride, magnesium, and phosphate—play an important role in making sure that the body works normally. When the level of electrolytes is not in proper balance, this can cause health problems for pregnant women and their babies. It's important to talk to your health-care provider if you have nausea and vomiting during pregnancy.

What can you do?

- When you first wake up, eat a few crackers or some dry toast, and then rest for 15 minutes.
- Get up slowly.
- Do not lie down right after eating.
- Eat small meals or snacks often so your stomach does not feel empty.
- Drink small amounts of fluids often during the day. Avoid drinking fluids during meals.
- Most pregnant women need more sleep during the first three months of pregnancy. Take a nap during the day.
- You may need to take time off work and get help and support from friends and family.

Taking medicine to control nausea and vomiting

DO NOT take over-the-counter medicines or herbal remedies when you are pregnant without talking to your health-care provider. Diclectin is the only prescription medication approved by Health Canada for the treatment of nausea and vomiting in pregnancy. It has been proven to have no harmful effects on babies.

To learn more about taking medications and herbal products when you are pregnant, visit the Motherisk Program's website at www.motherisk.org.

Acupressure and acupuncture treatments

These treatments have helped many pregnant women control their nausea and vomiting. About 30% of women find that the treatments relieve their symptoms. A person trained in this system will stimulate a

---

TIPS TO HELP SETTLE YOUR STOMACH

- **Avoid warm places;** *feeling hot can make your nausea worse.*
- **Eat smaller amounts** *of food and eat often.*
- **Sniff fresh lemons,** *drink lemonade, or eat slices of watermelon.*
- **Eat salty potato chips** *before a meal.*
- **Get acupressure or acupuncture treatments** *to help control nausea and vomiting.*
- **Avoid spicy, fried, or fatty foods.**
- **Avoid caffeine** *found in coffee, tea, and some carbonated (bubbly) drinks.*
- **Avoid brushing your teeth right after meals.**
- **Avoid smells that make you feel nauseous,** *such as cooking odours or perfume. Get your partner to prepare meals if possible.*
- *Find opportunities to* **increase rest times.**
- **Eat food cold** *so that the smell does not make you feel nauseous.*
- **Avoid drinking fluids during meals.**

Parasites are all around us. Most will not harm us or our unborn children. Then there is toxoplasmosis—a disease caused by a tiny parasite that lives in one animal and is passed on to other animals through its bowel movements (feces). As many as half of the people in the world have been exposed to this parasite. Although it is rare for an adult to have any symptoms when they come in contact with the parasite, there is a small risk of birth defects in a baby born to a pregnant woman exposed to the parasite during her pregnancy.

To be safe, you should avoid eating undercooked meat, chicken, or wild game when you are pregnant. Wear rubber gloves when you handle raw meat or chicken. If you have a cat, ask someone else to change the litter box so you are not exposed to this parasite. If you must do the job yourself:

- *wear gloves*
- *do not inhale the dust from the litter box*
- *wash your hands well when you have finished.*

Also, you should avoid digging in a garden or lawn where cats may have had bowel movements.

certain point on your forearm. Bracelets used for sea sickness (Seaband) also work on the same acupressure point.

Tender, painful breasts

You may want to get a good support bra and wear it all the time, even at night. Make sure it fits properly and that it has full, rounded cups with wide shoulder straps NOT made of elastic. You can also apply body cream.

Feeling tired

During the first few months of pregnancy, you may feel very tired. Do not worry—it's normal to feel this way. Many things are happening inside your body. First, your metabolism has increased, which consumes a lot of your energy. Second, one of the pregnancy hormones (progesterone) has the effect of making women feel sleepy.

The best advice is: do not try to fight the way you feel. Pay attention to your body and when you feel you need to rest or take a nap, just do it! Many women who "never nap" find themselves needing a little daytime rest. If you work outside the home, try to find a quiet place to relax and close your eyes when you have breaks. If this is impossible, plan to lie down as soon as you get home from work.

Headaches

Headaches are quite common during pregnancy. In most cases, there is no reason for alarm. However, if you have headaches all the time, or if they are very severe (cause blurred vision, nausea, or spots to appear in front of your eyes), you should contact your health-care provider.

If you have a headache:

- Lie down in a dark, cool room.
- Place a cool cloth on your forehead.

- Ask your partner for a neck and back massage.
- Try to eat small meals often. Sometimes, the headache is linked to low blood sugar, especially if you have a feeling of nausea and do not feel like eating.
- ***Do not use any pain medicine*** until you talk about it with your health-care provider.

The need to urinate often

Have you found yourself going to the bathroom more often lately? This is normal during early pregnancy because:

- your growing uterus is putting pressure on your bladder
- your kidneys are producing more urine

You may notice that, even though your bladder feels full, you only pass a little urine. Also, the pressure may cause urine to leak out when you move or cough. Kegel exercises may help (see page 50). However, if you feel any pain when you urinate, you may have an infection and you should talk to your health-care provider.

Light bleeding or spotting

Many women have a small amount of harmless spotting early in their pregnancy. They go on to give birth to healthy babies. But if you have any bleeding at all, you should take it seriously and get in touch with your health-care provider. If the bleeding persists and is heavier than a period—especially if it is associated with cramps—you may be at risk of a miscarriage. Seek emergency treatment right away.

Transport Canada has advised Canadians that the best way to protect an unborn child in a car crash is to protect the mother. Pregnant women should always wear the lap and shoulder seat belt.

- *The lap belt should be snug and low over the pelvic bones and not pressing against the soft stomach area.*

- *The shoulder belt should be worn across the chest.*

When worn the correct way, the seat belt will not harm the baby.

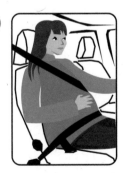

Source: Keep Kids Safe: Car Time 1-2-3-4, Transport Canada (TP 13511) www.tc.gc.ca/ roadsafety/tp/tp13511/tips.htm. Reproduced with the permission of the Minister of Public Works and Government Services Canada (2008).

Fainting

Feeling faint is common during pregnancy. It may be caused by a mix of:

- higher hormone levels
- changes to your circulation system
- low blood sugar levels

If you feel light-headed, try eating something sweet or have small nutritious snacks between meals. When you feel faint, sit down and put your head between your knees. Loosen any tight clothing and place a cool, wet cloth on your forehead or on the back of your neck. If the feeling does not go away, contact your health-care provider.

Your emotions during pregnancy

Taking care of your physical health is an important part of having a healthy pregnancy. But it's only one part. You also need to take care of your mental health.

When you are pregnant, it is normal to have mood swings. One minute you can be feeling happy about being pregnant, and the next you might find yourself worried and stressed out about the health of your baby or what will happen once the baby is born. The hormones that support your pregnancy and your baby also affect your moods. While some women may be moody all the way through their pregnancy, these highs and lows are most common between the 6th and 10th weeks and then again in the third trimester when your body is getting ready for labour and the baby's birth.

Here are some tips to help you take care of your emotional health when you are pregnant:

- Stay active and eat well.
- Take time to relax and rest.

- Avoid stressful situations and people.
- Share your thoughts and feelings with someone you trust.

Abuse during pregnancy

One in 12 women in Canada is a victim of physical violence. Physical abuse during pregnancy can hurt both the mother and her unborn baby. It may even cause her baby to be born too early or too small. Some unborn babies have died because of abuse suffered by their mothers.

If you are pregnant and are a victim of physical abuse, you probably feel very alone. You need help now.

No one deserves to be abused. Sometimes, abuse in a family can leave a woman feeling ashamed. She may feel that the abuse is her fault. If this is how you feel, please ask for help. Talk to your health-care provider, who will support you and help you find the community resources you need.

If you would like to learn more about abuse, and places you can call or visit for help, visit the website www.shelternet.ca or call the (S.O.S.) Domestic Violence 24-hour hotline at 1-800-363-9010.

Types of abuse that women suffer

There are many different kinds of abuse. But they all harm a pregnant woman and her growing baby in some way. If you live with abuse, be aware that it is not your fault and you can get help. Talk to your health-care provider if you are living with any of these kinds of abuse.

ARE YOU IN AN ABUSIVE RELATIONSHIP?

☐ *Do you solve disagreements with fighting?*

☐ *Do you feel frightened by what your partner says or does?*

☐ *Have you ever been hit, pushed, shoved, or slapped by your partner?*

☐ *Has your partner ever been mean to you or made you feel worthless or stupid?*

☐ *Have you ever been forced to have sex against your will?*

If you have answered yes to any of these questions, discuss this with your health-care provider or someone who can help.

 WHEN THE ONE WHO LOVES YOU HURTS YOU

CYCLE OF VIOLENCE

I'm Sorry
Romance
Stage

Tension
Builds

Explosive Event

Types of Abuse	
Physical abuse	*Slapping, punching, kicking, biting, shoving, and choking.*
Verbal abuse	*Constant criticism, blaming, false accusations, name calling, threats of violence toward you or the people or things you care about.*
Social abuse	*Isolating a woman from her family and friends.*
Sexual abuse	*Forcing a woman to be part of sexual activity.*
Emotional or psychosocial abuse	*Making a woman feel afraid, harassing a woman, being very jealous, trying to control a woman, making her feel isolated, threatening a woman.*
Environmental abuse	*Making a woman feel afraid in her own home by destroying property or things she owns.*
Financial abuse	*Stopping a woman from having control over money or spending, or exploiting her economically.*
Religious or spiritual abuse	*Making fun of a woman's beliefs, or using beliefs to manipulate her.*

Source: A Handbook for Health and Social Service Professionals Responding to Abuse During Pregnancy (1999), p.1, www.phac-aspc.gc.ca/ncfv-cnivf/familyviolence/pdfs/pregnancy_e.pdf, Public Health Agency of Canada. Reproduced with the permission of the Minister of Public Works and Government Services Canada, 2008.

Coping with stress and finding support

Everyone has some stress in their life, but having too much stress is not healthy, especially during pregnancy. Research shows that stress during pregnancy may be linked to preterm birth and low birth weight in babies.

The amount of support you receive from the people around you can have a direct effect on how much stress you feel during your pregnancy. If you receive very little support, you may feel lonely and depressed.

Although pregnancy is a joyous time for most couples, the changes and adjustments can sometimes cause strain in your relationship and increase your stress level. If you are not in a relationship, you may be feeling stressed about being all alone. Events you did not expect may happen even during pregnancy. This can also increase your stress levels.

If you find that your stress level is rising, look for community resources that can help you find ways to reduce your stress and deal with challenges.

Ways to reduce your stress

Women with too much stress need to learn healthy ways to deal with it. Here are some tips:

1. **Talk about it.** Share the joys, problems, and worries of pregnancy with someone close to you. This can make your pregnancy seem less stressful. If, for some reason, you do not have the support of your partner, try to spend time with other people whose company you enjoy.

2. **Learn about pregnancy and childbirth.** Attend prenatal classes and meet other women going through pregnancy, too. The breathing and concentration exercises you will learn for childbirth can help you relax now. By knowing what to expect and being prepared, you can reduce any worry you may be feeling about the birth itself. Working with your health-care provider and support person to prepare a birth plan may help, too. (Read about birth plans on pages 101 and 102.)

3. **Get active.** Exercise is a proven way to lift your spirits and reduce stress.

4. **Rest and relax.** Make sure you are sleeping enough. Learn other ways to rest and relax. Your public library will have books and audiotapes about reducing stress and learning to relax.

Miscarriages do happen

Perhaps the most stressful thing that can happen in a pregnancy is a miscarriage. They occur in 15 to 20% of pregnancies and they happen most often during the first eight weeks. BUT, a number of miscarriages take place before a woman misses a menstrual cycle, or is even aware that she is pregnant.

The cause of miscarriage is often unknown. We think it is the body's natural response to an embryo that is not growing properly and would not be able to survive. Although the 15 to 20% rate for miscarriages seems to be high, it includes those that happen in the very early days of a pregnancy.

It's important for all pregnant women to take any vaginal bleeding seriously. You should also know that 20% of mothers have some bleeding before the 20th week and that about half of these pregnancies will continue without further problems.

Bleeding may begin in the uterus, cervix, or vagina. You should seek medical attention if the bleeding soaks a thick sanitary pad every hour, over a period of two hours.

Although a miscarriage does not affect most women's future fertility or their ability to carry a child to full term, doctors suggest waiting for at least one regular menstrual cycle before trying to become pregnant again. Also, emotional healing is just as important as physical healing. Any woman who has a miscarriage should expect to feel a range of emotions as well as physical discomforts. Grieving allows the mother to begin the healing process, which is unique for each person.

My pregnancy journal
10 to 16 weeks

This visit takes place about four weeks after your first appointment. In most cases, you will not have a complete physical exam. You should expect to be weighed and have your blood pressure taken. Your health-care provider will check the growth of your uterus and may also check your baby's heart rate.

At this visit, you and your health-care provider will discuss the results of any tests that were ordered last time. You may also talk about any other testing or actions that may be recommended.

As with every prenatal visit, you should be prepared to tell your health-care provider about any concerns or questions you may have. Filling out this section of the handbook can help you prepare for each visit. Bring this handbook with you. Then you will have notes from your last visit, as well as a list of questions that have occurred to you in the meantime.

If possible, it's a good idea for your partner or support person (close friend, mother, or other family member) to attend a visit to your health-care provider at least once. This will give them a chance to meet the person who is caring for you and voice any concerns or questions they may have.

MY DUE DATE:

KEEPING TRACK OF MY PROGRESS

Date:

Week of pregnancy:

Blood pressure:

Weight:

Fetal heart rate:

THINGS TO DISCUSS WITH MY HEALTH-CARE PROVIDER:

• *What are the benefits and risks of genetic testing?*

• *What advice do you have to help control nausea and vomiting?*

• *How much weight should I gain?*

• *Am I eating the right foods?*

• *Is it okay to have sex?*

• *Am I doing too much or too little exercise?*

• *I have concerns about abuse in my relationship.*

• *What are Kegel exercises?*

• *Other concerns:*

My test results:

Hemoglobin: (Normal 110–120 mg/L)

Blood type:

Immunity to: Rubella: Yes/No

　　　　　　　Chicken pox: Yes/No

Other results:

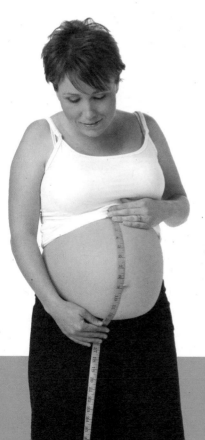

CHAPTER THREE

Gentle growth:
the second trimester

MEASURING YOUR BABY'S GROWTH

A routine part of your prenatal check-up is a measurement called SFH, which stands for Symphysis Fundal Height. Your health-care provider will make a physical measurement on your abdomen that tells you how well your baby is growing.

The SFH is the distance from your pubic bone to where the top of your uterus bulges from your belly — this part of the uterus is called the fundus. The fundus usually reaches to the top of the pubic bone by about the 12th week of pregnancy. It reaches under your rib cage by the 36th week. Between the 18th and 30th weeks, the height of the fundus (in centimetres) is close to the age of the baby in weeks.

Introduction

Congratulations on reaching the second trimester. Your pregnancy is considered well-established and there is a much lower chance of having a miscarriage. This trimester will last from the 15th to the 25th weeks, or from your fourth month to halfway through your sixth month. You will begin to feel more like you did before pregnancy began. Morning sickness and minor discomforts that you felt during the first trimester should be behind you.

You will likely feel new discomforts, but many women enjoy this part of their pregnancy because:

- *they are comfortable with their size;*
- *they like the way they look.*

Your baby will be growing at a rapid pace, and will soon be big enough for you to feel the rolls, somersaults, and kicks. Guess what? Babies like to exercise. The second trimester is when you will have an ultrasound. This will give you a sense of what your baby looks like.

In this chapter, we will talk about:

- *preterm labour and birth,*
- *work,*
- *swelling, and*
- *backaches.*

We will also provide places for you to keep track of new information about you and your baby.

Your changing body

During your second trimester, you will probably feel calmer and more settled. The placenta, which has been developing in your uterus, has taken over most of the hormone production that sustains your pregnancy (see page 4 to learn more about the placenta). It is also the place where the baby's umbilical cord attaches to your uterus. At this time during pregnancy, your hormone levels should begin to even out.

You will also notice that your body's shape and size will begin to change. With these changes will come more physical discomforts that are linked to many factors, not just the baby's size. You may worry if your friends or family say that you seem "small" or look "large." Try not to worry about these comments. If you have been having regular prenatal visits, you will know that your baby is growing just fine.

So what determines your size during pregnancy? Your normal height, weight, and build—before you were pregnant—and whether or not this is your first pregnancy will have an impact on how your body grows and changes. Short women tend to look bigger. Large-boned or taller women tend to look smaller. Second-time mothers tend to have bigger bellies because the muscles of the abdomen and uterus were stretched before.

The colour of your skin (pigmentation) may be different with your changing hormones. You may develop a brownish, vertical line down the middle of your belly. This is called the *linea nigra*. Some women develop brownish, uneven marks around their eyes and over the nose and cheeks. These marks usually go away when hormone levels return to normal after your baby's birth.

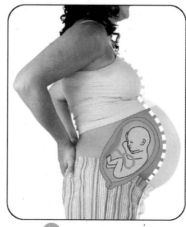

▶ *2nd trimester*

As your breasts begin to get ready to feed your baby, you may notice a little **colostrum** leaking from the nipples. Colostrum is the clear sticky fluid your breasts produce for your baby's first feedings, before they begin to produce breast milk. It contains many important antibodies to protect your baby against infections.

As a way to get ready for birth, hormones in your body will soften the ligaments and cartilage in your pelvis and back.

Your growing baby

Wait until you see the ultrasound of your baby—at about the 18th week. You will see that your fetus is really looking like a baby—perfectly formed with all body systems in place, working well, and beginning to mature. The skin is red because the blood vessels are close to the surface. Some fat is starting to form under the skin, and a thick coating of a white, cheese-like substance called **vernix** covers the entire body.

The eyelids open and close by 26 weeks. The fingernails are full length and many babies have a visible hairline. Eyebrows and scalp hair become visible at the end of the 20th week and by 24 weeks you can even see the eyelashes. The amniotic sac is filled with a large amount of fluid that contains both nutrients for growth and small amounts of the baby's urine. The umbilical cord is thick, strong, and very firm, which helps prevent knots from forming.

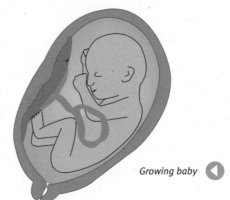

Growing baby

Preterm labour

Preterm labour means that your labour begins too early—weeks before the baby is supposed to be born. Not all women understand how important it is to carry a baby to full term. Some women hope for a premature baby, thinking it will be easier to give birth to a smaller baby.

Premature babies are more fragile and preterm labour is one of the most common problems in pregnancy. It causes 75% of all deaths in newborns with no other major problems. Being born early can cause them to have life-long challenges. In general, the earlier a baby is born, the more severe the problems. Babies born before the 25th week usually do not survive without problems.

It's important to know the early signs of preterm labour because sometimes it can be stopped or delayed. The sooner you notice preterm labour, the more time there is to give medicine that can help the baby, and to treat any of the conditions that might be causing preterm labour.

What causes preterm labour?

We do not really know the causes. About half of all preterm labours begin for no obvious reason, to women who seem to be having a normal pregnancy. However, certain things seem to increase a woman's chances of going into early labour.

As you've been reading this handbook, you have learned that the best way to have a healthy pregnancy and deliver a healthy baby is to avoid risks and take care of your health.

In France, one long-term study showed that the rate of premature births dropped when:

- There was public education about preterm labour and the importance of healthy full-term babies to society as a whole.

ARE YOU AT RISK FOR PRETERM LABOUR?

As you read this list, check off any statements that apply to you.

☐ *I have no regular prenatal care.*

☐ *I have high blood pressure.*

☐ *There is a lot of stress in my life.*

☐ *My partner or someone else I love abuses me in a physical or emotional way.*

☐ *I am pregnant with more than one fetus.*

☐ *A previous baby of mine was born too early.*

☐ *I weigh less than 45.5 kg (100 lbs).*

☐ *I have a chronic illness.*

☐ *I smoke.*

☐ *I quit smoking cigarettes, but not until after my 32nd week of pregnancy.*

☐ *I work long hours (more than 8 hours a day) or do shift work.*

☐ *My work is very physically demanding (strenuous).*

If you checked off one or more boxes, you are at risk for preterm labour. You should talk to your health-care provider to learn how to help prevent preterm labour.

PRETERM LABOUR CAN HAPPEN
TO ANYONE, BUT THERE ARE WAYS
TO HELP PREVENT IT. HERE
ARE SOME OF THE SIGNS OF
PRETERM LABOUR:

- *Regular contractions of the uterus before your baby is due*
- *Low dull backache*
- *A feeling of pressure in the lower abdomen, the pelvis, or the lower back.*

LEARN THE SIGNS OF PRETERM
LABOUR. ACT RIGHT AWAY
AND FIND A WAY TO GO TO THE
NEAREST HOSPITAL SAFELY
IF YOU EXPERIENCE ANY OF
THESE SYMPTOMS:

- *Bleeding*
- *Leaking or a gush of fluid from your vagina*
- *Pain in your abdomen that you cannot explain*
- *A decrease in your baby's movement*
- *Unusual and constant headaches*
- *Blurred vision or spots before your eyes*
- *Feeling dizzy*
- *Dull pain in your lower back that does not go away*
- *Being in a motor vehicle accident.*

- Special seats on buses and special parking spots were set aside for pregnant women.
- Pregnant women were encouraged to keep their own pregnancy record (much like this book).

Here are some of the risk factors for preterm labour and tips on how you can reduce your risk:

Smoking

It's best not to smoke during pregnancy and it's never too late to quit. It's still good for your baby if you quit smoking before you reach 32 weeks. (Read the section on smoking on page 31.)

Working too hard

Working long hours, doing very physical work, and being tired all the time can lead to a preterm birth. (Read the section about physical work on page 84.)

Physical and emotional abuse

When someone hurts you, they can also hurt your unborn baby. Even emotional abuse can lead to a preterm birth by raising your stress levels. If you are being abused by your partner or someone you love, seek help by calling a family crisis centre in your area. (Read the section on abuse during pregnancy on page 67.)

Incompetent cervix

This is a condition in which the cervix opens (dilates) too soon. The cervix is supposed to open when the baby is full-term and ready to be born, but in rare situations, the cervix can open too soon and cause premature birth. The mother may be unaware of the condition, but the problem can be discovered during a vaginal exam, or when the size of the cervix is measured during an ultrasound. Sometimes, the problem can be treated by sewing the cervix closed with a "drawstring" stitch and removing the stitches when the baby is full-term.

Fibroids

Large fibroids—growths in the muscle wall of the uterus—can push the uterus out of its natural shape and can cause pain and preterm labour. If the fibroids grow large enough to deform the uterus and are found before you become pregnant, they may be removed. Small fibroids usually don't cause problems during pregnancy.

Bleeding during the second trimester

A small amount of bleeding can happen if the placenta starts to pull away from the lining of the uterus before labour starts. But do not assume that you know the cause of the bleeding, even if you have been treated for bleeding before. Every time you bleed, you need to see your health-care provider right away. Always contact your health-care provider if you notice any bleeding.

Abdominal surgery during pregnancy

Sometimes a pregnant woman may need abdominal surgery (for example, if she has a health crisis with her appendix). However, you should avoid any other kinds of surgery that are not essential until after the baby is born.

Common infections during pregnancy

Infections of the vagina, cervix, kidney, and bladder are common during pregnancy and must be treated. A bladder or kidney infection may cause you pain when you urinate, or may make you feel like you need to pass urine often but then you produce only a small amount. The signs of an infection in your vagina or cervix include unusual discharge from your vagina, pain in your pelvis or groin area, or a fever. If you suspect an infection, contact your health-care provider.

WHEN SOMETHING GOES WRONG

- *Call the hospital and talk to a nurse in the case room.*

  Phone number:

- *Call your health-care provider.*

  Phone number:

Being underweight during pregnancy

Treatment depends on the cause of the problem. Sometimes this problem can be helped just by eating healthy food on a regular basis. Talk to your health-care provider if you are concerned that you may be underweight.

Placenta previa

This is a problem where the placenta implants and grows over the opening of the cervix (where the baby must come out). This can cause heavy bleeding during labour. In most cases, the problem is found during routine ultrasound testing. The woman may be confined to bed rest for the last few weeks of pregnancy and the baby is usually born by Caesarean section before labour has a chance to begin.

Preterm rupture of the membranes

This is when the sac of amniotic fluid breaks or leaks before your baby reaches full term. It may be linked to infections in the uterus, but research has not yet revealed the cause. If your membranes rupture early, treatment depends on how much amniotic fluid is lost and how close to your due date you are. If this happens to you, contact your health-care provider right away.

Gestational hypertension (high blood pressure caused by pregnancy)

This can be treated in different ways, depending on how serious it is. (Read more about it on page 97.)

Chronic illness in the mother

Some illnesses (such as diabetes or high blood pressure) may become more serious during pregnancy. In some cases, the only way to stop the condition from getting worse is to deliver the baby. Sometimes, the labour will begin too early on its own; in other cases, the labour needs to be started (induced) by medical means.

Preterm babies

While only about 7 out of 100 babies are born preterm, they face more problems than other babies and may even die. Labour should not happen between weeks 15 and 25 of the second trimester. Normally, labour begins sometime after your 37th week of pregnancy and before the end of your 41st week. If labour starts before you reach your 37th week, your labour is called "preterm."

The main reason premature babies have problems is that their body organs are not ready to work all by themselves—they are not mature enough. For example, a baby's lungs are not usually ready to begin breathing until close to the end of the pregnancy. Babies born before their lungs can breathe on their own may suffer mild to severe breathing problems that could last a lifetime. An immature stomach and bowels can lead to feeding problems. When your baby's immune system is not able to work on its own, your baby is more likely to get infections.

Premature babies can also develop problems with their eyes and ears. Because their blood vessels are so close to the skin's surface and they have very little fat under their skin, they are redder and thinner than those of full-term babies. Without fat deposits, premature babies have problems staying warm. Premature babies are also more likely to be delivered by Caesarean section. When you are pregnant, it is best for you and your unborn child to do all that you can to prevent your baby from being born before he reaches full term.

If you are pregnant with twins or multiples, you and your health-care provider will work together to ensure that your babies are born as close to full-term as possible. To learn more about multiple births, see Chapter Two.

Labour and checking for preterm labour

Labour begins when your uterus starts to get tight (contract) at regular intervals. As labour begins and your body prepares for your baby's travel down the birth canal:

- The cervix will begin to thin out (efface) and open up (dilate).
- The mucous plug that formed during pregnancy to protect the entrance of your uterus may come loose. This will produce a bloody discharge called a "show."
- Your "water" may break—this is when the sac filled with amniotic fluid that surrounds your baby breaks open suddenly.

The only way to know for sure if you are in preterm labour is to be checked by a nurse, a midwife, or a doctor. They will be able to tell what type of contractions you are having and if the cervix is opening. During this check-up, your health-care provider will give you a full examination. They may also use an ultrasound to learn more about the size and position of your baby, as well as to measure the length of your cervix. When the cervix gets shorter, this is a sign that preterm labour could be starting. Many hospitals have a special test that involves checking for a substance in the vaginal fluid that shows whether a woman is in preterm labour or not.

If your labour has been confirmed as real labour (not false labour), and depending on how close to full-term you are, you and your health-care provider will need to decide whether to try to stop your labour or let it continue. They will also likely advise you to take medication to help prepare the baby's lungs for breathing. In most cases, it's better for the baby to have as much time as possible to grow and develop inside your uterus.

What you can do to prevent preterm labour

Here are the main things you can do to try to prevent your baby from being born too soon.

Quit smoking

Try to understand why you smoke and seek help to learn other ways of dealing with the reasons for smoking. Find out about Quit Smoking programs in your community. Ask your health-care provider about programs to help you quit.

Eat properly

Talk to a registered dietitian about your eating habits. Plan your meals around the basic food groups and avoid junk food. Drink plenty of milk. Make sure you get enough protein and that you eat foods rich in omega-3 fatty acids (see page 23).

Get help for abuse

You have a right to feel safe. If you are being abused, call your local women's shelter and ask where you can go for help.

Get plenty of rest

Plan ahead to make sure you get time to rest every day. Do not feel guilty about resting. It is very important during pregnancy.

Learn ways to reduce stress

Talk to people you trust about how you feel. Learn ways to relax, such as meditation and self-massage. Find your own healthy ways to reduce stress. Join a yoga class if you think you will enjoy it.

IS MY WORK TOO PHYSICALLY DEMANDING?

As you read this list, check off any statements that are true for you.

When I am at work . . .

- [ ] *I stoop or bend over more than ten times each hour.*
- [ ] *I climb a ladder more than three times during an eight-hour shift.*
- [ ] *I stand for more than four hours at one time.*
- [ ] *I climb stairs more than three times per shift.*
- [ ] *I work more than 40 hours per week.*
- [ ] *I work shift work.*
- [ ] *I will need to lift more than 23 kg (50 lbs) after the 20th week of my pregnancy.*
- [ ] *I will need to lift more than 11 kg (24 lbs) after 24 weeks.*
- [ ] *I will need to stoop, bend, or climb ladders after my 28th week.*
- [ ] *I will need to lift heavy items after my 30th week.*
- [ ] *I will need to stand still for more than 30 minutes of every hour after 32 weeks.*

If you checked off any of these boxes, parts of your work may not be right for you while you are pregnant. Your health-care provider may strongly suggest that you change the work you do until after your baby is born. (Read more about work during pregnancy on pages 30 and 85.)

Avoid very physical work

Read about what work is too physical and demanding (strenuous) for a pregnant woman (see sidebar). Avoid doing these things during pregnancy.

Avoid intense exercise

Even if you are physically fit, you should not make your workouts more intense during certain times of your pregnancy. (Read more about this on page 46.)

Learn the signs of preterm labour

Prenatal classes offered by your hospital or community centre are an excellent way to learn about the signs of preterm labour. (Read more about the signs on page 78.) Talk to your health-care provider.

Learn what to do if you think you are in preterm labour

Talk to your health-care provider about what you should do and write down the phone numbers of people you should call. (See page 82.)

Visit your health-care provider regularly

This is one of the most important things you can do to prevent preterm labour. Doing so gives your health-care provider a chance to find or prevent any problems that might cause your baby to be born early.

Gestational diabetes

For some women, pregnancy hormones change the way their bodies use insulin. They may then develop a type of diabetes that only happens during pregnancy. It is called ***gestational diabetes***. Your health-care provider may order a test for gestational diabetes at around 24 to 28 weeks. Most pregnant women with this problem will be able to control their blood sugar levels by following a special diet and exercising. A small number may require insulin by injection to control their blood sugar levels. For most, the condition goes away after the baby is born, but some may go on to develop diabetes later in life. With knowledge, good control, and professional care by a health-care team, most women with gestational diabetes have a safe pregnancy and a healthy baby.

(For information about the special needs of women who have Type 1 or insulin-dependent diabetes before they become pregnant, see pages 60 to 62.)

About fetal movement

Babies move their arms and legs to exercise and to find a more comfortable position. If you are pregnant for the first time, you may not feel your baby move until about your 19th week. If this is a second (or later) child, you will usually begin to feel movement sooner, at around the 17th week. From that point on, you should feel your baby move at different times of the day, every day. Keep in mind that babies sleep at certain times of the day, and will be more active at other times. You may be asked to keep track of your baby's movements by counting the number of kicks you feel. (See page 96 for how to count movements.)

About work

In most normal pregnancies, the type of work you do is not usually a problem. However, strenuous work or standing up for a long time have been linked to a slight rise in problems such as low-birth-weight

---

MATERNITY AND PARENTAL LEAVES

Each province has different rules for the length of maternity and parental leaves. For more information about what applies to you, see the Human Resources and Skills Development Canada website:

www.hrsdc.gc.ca

Pregnant women can have access to government programs for maternity leave. If the need arises, and if required, your health-care provider can advise you to stop work because of concerns about your health. You should still get paid while you are absent.

While bed rest may be recommended for some conditions during pregnancy, it can also lead to problems, such as:

- *blood clots (mainly in the legs);*

- *loss of muscle strength (muscular atrophy);*

- *skin sores (lesions);*

- *emotional distress;*

- *depression.*

Sometimes these problems continue even after the baby is born. If your health-care provider puts you on bed rest, you can use the bed rest exercises in the sidebar on page 87. They may help you to avoid or reduce some of the challenges listed above. You may be able to increase your flexibility and range of motion, and the exercises may even help prepare you for labour.

babies, preterm labour, and miscarriage. To find out if your work is too demanding for a pregnant woman, answer the questions in the sidebar on page 84.

You also might be at risk if you work with certain chemicals. Governments have set rules to limit human exposure to toxic chemicals. To find out more about environmental hazards and pregnancy, see the Motherisk website www.motherisk.org and consult government health and safety regulations.

Common discomforts during the second trimester

Backaches

Your growing belly will make you lean back to find your centre of gravity, which then strains your back muscles. The weight of the uterus in your pelvis, combined with joint movement and joint softening, can also give you backaches during pregnancy. To prevent backaches:

- always try to sit up straight
- avoid wearing high heels
- lift heavy objects by bending your legs and crouching rather than bending from your waist
- avoid standing for long periods of time

Your health-care provider may suggest that you see a licensed massage therapist, physiotherapist, or chiropractor. Yoga, stretching, and learning new ways to relax may help too. Read about pelvic tilt exercises on page 50. Be sure to change your body position often and take time to lie down, put your feet up, and relax. Try using heat, ice packs, or massages to ease the pain.

Constipation

During pregnancy, your food moves more slowly through your bowels. This slowing down can lead to *constipation* (irregular or difficult bowel movements). If you are taking iron supplements, they can cause constipation (and may turn your stools black). To help keep the stool (bodily waste) from becoming dry and hard, you should drink at least eight glasses of fluid (juice, water, or milk) daily. Getting regular exercise and eating plenty of fibre will help too. Foods that are high in fibre include:

- ground flaxseed
- whole grain breads and cereals
- raw vegetables
- raw and dried fruit
- psyllium

If needed, your health-care provider may suggest a bulk-forming agent or stool softener.

Hemorrhoids

Many expectant mothers will develop *hemorrhoids* (swollen veins in the rectum). Hemorrhoids often flare up during pregnancy because your growing uterus places a lot of pressure on these veins. If a woman strains to have a bowel movement because she has hard stools, the hemorrhoids become worse, and may push out around the anal opening. Sometimes they are painful and bleed. Try to eat foods that will reduce constipation (see above). Your health-care provider may suggest ointments to help shrink the hemorrhoids.

Urinary tract infections (UTIs)

The **urinary tract** is made up of the kidneys, ureters, bladder, and urethra. Infections in the urinary tract are common during pregnancy.

Here's how the urinary tract works:

- Urine is made in the two kidneys.
- From each kidney, urine drips down tubes (ureters) into the bladder.

LEG EXTENSIONS (CAN BE DONE LYING ON YOUR SIDE OR INCLINED ON YOUR BACK)

Hook your hands on the back of one leg and extend the leg out. Exhale while you hold the leg straight for two seconds. Then, bend your other leg. Repeat, using the other leg. Go back and forth between the left and right legs for one to three sets (of 20) at least three times daily. Complete this exercise by holding your leg extended for a count of 12 to stretch the hamstring muscle.

UPPER BODY BED REST COMBO (USING A LOW-TENSION EXERCISE BAND)

Get into an inclined position. If you are at home, use pillows to prop yourself up.

Bend your knees slightly and hook the middle of the exercise band around the bottom of your feet. Holding the band, lift your arms above your head (shoulder press). Then, lower and lift your arms to the side (side raise). Then, lower and finish the set by curling the band toward your biceps for a biceps curl.

THINGS YOU CAN DO:

- *Avoid lying down for one to two hours after eating.*
- *Raise the head of your bed (30 degrees or 6 inches).*
- *Wear loose clothing, especially around the waist.*
- *Avoid exercise after eating.*
- *Eat smaller amounts of food more often.*
- *Eat slowly and chew your food well.*
- *Drink fluids between meals rather than during meals.*

FOODS TO AVOID:

- *fatty or deep-fried foods*
- *rich desserts, such as cheesecake*
- *spicy foods*
- *onions and garlic*
- *citrus fruit, such as oranges, grapefruit, and lemons*
- *tomatoes*
- *spearmint and peppermint*
- *coffee and tea*
- *chocolate*
- *carbonated beverages (soda pop, drinks with bubbles)*

• When the bladder is full, urine leaves the body through an important tube called the urethra.

Infections of the urethra can sometimes be hard to detect. The common signs of an infection in your lower urinary tract (bladder) are:

• pain when you urinate
• having to urinate more often than usual
• only passing urine in very small amounts—even though you feel like your bladder is full

This kind of infection can be treated easily with antibiotics.

An upper urinary tract infection (which involves the kidneys) is more serious. It can cause chills, fever, nausea, vomiting, backache, pain in the side of your body, and pain in your lower abdomen.

Women who are prone to either lower or upper UTIs should be very careful when they are pregnant. UTIs are thought to be one of the causes of preterm labour. Be sure to inform your health-care provider about flu-like symptoms because it may, in fact, be more serious.

Indigestion and heartburn

If you have a burning feeling at the back of your throat, lower in your food pipe (esophagus), or in your stomach, you may be suffering from indigestion. This is often caused by pregnancy hormones and the pressure of your growing uterus against your stomach.

It may help to:

• eat small amounts of food more often
• eat slowly
• chew your food well
• drink fluids between rather than during meals
• avoid caffeine and greasy, spicy foods that cause gas

- sit upright after a meal to give the food time to pass from the stomach into the intestine
- wear loose clothing

Only take antacids after speaking with your health-care provider. Antacids can cause a negative effect, where your stomach produces even more acids after the antacid wears off. As well, antacids that contain aluminum may make it hard to absorb certain minerals from food.

Groin pain

The round ligament that holds the uterus in place sometimes goes into spasms when it stretches as your baby grows. This stretching may feel like a stabbing pain on one or both sides of your lower belly, or it can feel like a dull ache. These pains seem to be most common in the second trimester. Pregnant women sometimes worry that groin pain is preterm labour. It may help to avoid turning your waist quickly. When you do feel pain, lean into it (bend toward the pain) to help relax the tension on the muscles. Lie down and get some rest. If the pain continues or gets worse—and if it does not go away when you change positions—go to the obstetrics ward of your hospital or visit your health-care provider.

Feeling dizzy when you are flat on your back

If you lie on your back, the blood supply to your brain may be reduced. This can make you feel light-headed and dizzy. It can happen because of pressure on the vena cava, one of the largest blood vessels in your body. It brings blood from the lower part of your body up to your heart. Because the vena cava runs right beside your spine, if your heavy uterus squeezes it against your spine, you may have less blood supply to your heart, lungs, and brain. Find a position—lying on either side of your body, or even on an incline—that makes you comfortable. Please do not worry about lying on your back, or feel that you must lie only on your

TIPS TO HELP REDUCE THE SWELLING IN YOUR LEGS, ANKLES, AND FEET:

- *Get regular exercise using your legs (e.g. swimming, walking, etc.).*

- *Do not cross your legs when you are seated.*

- *Wear support hose and avoid socks with tight bands of elastic around the top.*

- *Do not stand for too long.*

- *Raise your legs above the level of your heart as often as you can.*

- *Drink 8 glasses of fluids (juice, water, or milk) each day. This will help you avoid dehydration. How much you need to drink can depend on many factors, such as your activity level. At least 8 glasses a day would be a good beginning. If your urine is yellow (one sign of dehydration), increase your fluid intake. Your urine should be pale in colour.*

- *Do not remove salt from your diet.*

left side. Anything that makes you comfortable and lets you get some rest is what's best.

Swelling of your legs, ankles, and feet

A small amount of swelling in your legs, ankles, and feet is normal during pregnancy. This type of swelling builds up each day and should mostly disappear by the time you get up the next morning. It can be more of a problem if the weather is quite warm. Make sure you drink plenty of fluids (8 glasses a day) and do not remove salt from your diet, because your body needs some salt for day-to-day functions. If your hands or face swell, it may mean that you have a different, more serious problem, such as high blood pressure (see page 97).

Stretch marks

Many women get stretch marks—or streaks that are reddish—on their breasts, belly, and thighs during pregnancy. Nobody really knows if lotions and oils help reduce stretch marks, but many women rub oils (such as vitamin E oil or lanolin) on their bellies. Whether or not it works for stretch marks, the motion of rubbing your belly with lotions and oils will help both you and your unborn child relax. No harm can come from doing this.

Dry, itchy skin

Try not to use harsh soaps, because they tend to wash away the natural oils in your skin. If you must use soap, use one made with glycerine. Try not to lie in a tub of water for too long; this can also dry out your skin. Putting oil or an oatmeal-based softener in the bath will help. If you use bath oils, be careful not to slip when you get out of the tub. The oils can make the bathtub very slippery. After a bath or shower, apply body lotion to your damp skin. This will help keep your skin supple, soft, and moisturized.

My pregnancy journal
16 to 24 weeks

As was the case with the last prenatal visit, your examination will include weighing and measuring you and your baby.

At 16 to 18 weeks, your health-care provider may suggest a screening ultrasound test. The images from the ultrasound let your health-care provider measure the size of your baby, and help to confirm your baby's due date.

Date:

Week of pregnancy:

Blood pressure:

Weight:

Fetal heart rate:

THINGS TO DISCUSS WITH MY HEALTH-CARE PROVIDER:

• *Am I at risk for preterm labour?*

• *Is my work too physically demanding?*

• *Other concerns:*

My test results:

Gestational diabetes test: (Normal = 3.8–7.8 mmol/L)

Ultrasound results:

Other results:

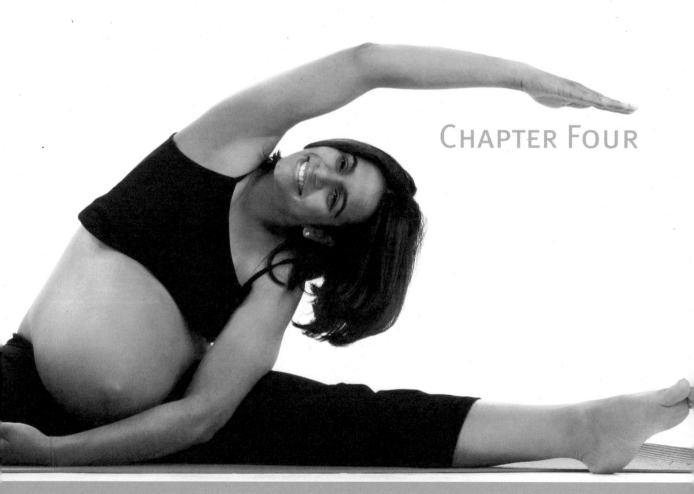

CHAPTER FOUR

The home stretch: the third trimester

Introduction

Welcome to your third trimester. After 25 weeks, you'll be looking forward to the arrival of your baby (and the end of your pregnancy). If you're starting to feel a bit anxious and tired—congratulations, you're right on schedule.

So, let's look ahead to the rest of this handbook and how it will help guide you through to the final stages of your pregnancy—and your baby's birth. Here in Chapter Four, we're going to give you a few more tips to make you aware of common problems such as hypertension (also known as high blood pressure). We will help you prepare a brief "birth plan" that will detail your needs when your baby decides to arrive (imagine that, a child with a mind of its own!).

During your last month of pregnancy, your prenatal visits will be more frequent. You should expect to see your health-care provider as often as once a week during the final month. Each visit will involve a check of your blood pressure, your urine, and the position of the baby. The goal will be to assess your general health and the health of your baby.

We won't cover the Big Day for a couple of chapters yet, but you'll be wondering what to expect in the hospital and this chapter will prepare you for the event. We also include a section on breastfeeding to help you to decide how to feed your baby.

You can peek ahead to the final four chapters, which will take you through the first few weeks of parenthood. The next two chapters will cover the final six weeks before the Big Day, and then the birth itself. After that, the following chapter will discuss YOU—and getting back to "normal." Finally, we'll offer a chapter of information that will help get you started with your new family member.

Your changing body

During your third trimester, you are going to become visibly pregnant. The top of your uterus will extend from above your navel to under your rib cage and your belly will stick out even further. This might make you feel more uncomfortable. You will feel pressure on your ribs and in your pelvis. Your abdominal muscles will feel stretched. You may feel sharp pains in your groin or vagina as your baby's head goes into the pelvis.

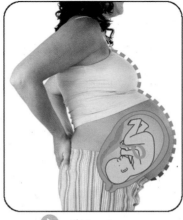

▶ *3rd trimester*

Your growing baby

Your baby was fully formed in the second trimester and will now keep growing in a steady way. At 25 to 26 weeks, the baby's weight will be between 700 and 900 grams (1-1/2 to 2 pounds). By 35 to 36 weeks, this same baby will weigh 2500 grams (5-1/2 pounds). By your due date, the weight will be between 3000 and 4000 grams (6-1/2 to 9 pounds).

Preterm birth is still a concern. Although all the organ systems are formed, they must still mature fully before they can function on their own. Between weeks 20 and 21, your baby's "breathing" movements become regular and between weeks 26 and 29, the baby would be able to breathe air if it were to be born. The baby's arms and legs are bent close to the body. Now, the uterus is starting to feel crowded. You should still feel active movement each day, although the fetus (like a newborn) has times when it is active, and when it is at rest.

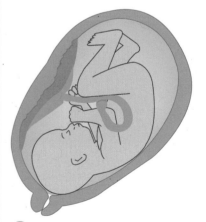

▶ *Growing baby*

Your prenatal care

Examinations will include more measurements of your weight and blood pressure, urine tests, and your baby's position and growth. Toward the end of the third trimester, you will likely have vaginal exams to make sure that your cervix is "ripening." This means it is getting itself ready for delivery.

You will be asked about your baby's movements. These details give your health-care provider important information about the baby's health. You may also be asked to do daily fetal movement counts (see below).

Your health-care provider may order other tests for your baby. Common tests that measure the well-being of a fetus are:

Counting the baby's movements: One of the best ways to know if your baby is healthy is to measure the amount of activity. You can do "movement counts" at home. The best time to do this is in the early evening while you are reclining (not lying down flat) in a comfortable position. Take some quiet time, and have a clock nearby. See how long it takes you to count six movements. If the count does not reach six movements in two hours, contact your health-care provider or hospital right away. It may be recommended that you have more testing.

You are the best judge of whether your baby is moving less often or in a new manner. Be aware that overdue babies feel very crowded and their movements may not feel as strong as they did earlier in the pregnancy. But no matter what, you should still feel movement throughout the day, every day. Your health-care provider may ask you to write down your baby's movement counts.

Ultrasound testing: An ultrasound helps your health-care provider monitor your baby's health by checking growth, movement, and the amount of amniotic fluid. The results of this test are often compared to any ultrasounds you had in the past.

Non-stress test: A non-stress test records your baby's heart rate. It may be done at your health-care provider's clinic or at the hospital. The rate is measured for 20 to 30 minutes. If the baby is healthy, the test will show that the baby's heart rate rises with movement.

Stripping the membranes

Your prenatal visits may also include some simple procedures such as "stripping" the membranes. You should also expect tests for possible problems such as hypertension (high blood pressure) and Group B Streptococcus (GBS).

Stripping the membranes is a simple procedure done to separate the amniotic sac membranes from the cervix, without breaking through the membranes. It helps your body get ready for the birth. It is a common and acceptable practice that helps to ripen the cervix and may help to prevent your pregnancy from being overdue. After talking about this procedure with you and getting your consent, your health-care provider will place a finger into your cervix (much like putting a finger into a small doughnut hole), and then circle the finger against the inside of the cervix to detach the membrane that is stuck to the sides. This routine procedure usually happens sometime after 38 weeks and can be performed in your health-care provider's office. After it is done, most women have a bit of cramping that lasts a short time, along with a small amount of pink discharge.

High blood pressure during pregnancy

High blood pressure, also known as hypertension, is fairly common during pregnancy. Your health-care provider will check your blood pressure often and may check for protein in your urine. You may also need to have some blood tests to see if your high blood pressure is a problem.

Your health-care provider will check for high blood pressure (greater than 140/90) and protein in your urine and will send you to the laboratory for blood work, and possibly for fetal monitoring.

During pregnancy, the most common types of high blood pressure are:

• Pre-existing hypertension (which appears before 20 weeks of pregnancy).
• Gestational hypertension (which develops after 20 weeks of pregnancy).

About 5 to 10% of pregnant women will develop a form of pregnancy-related hypertension known as pre-eclampsia, or toxemia. When this happens, your blood pressure is high and you may also have protein in your urine. You may be feeling symptoms such as severe headaches, pain around your liver, irritability, swelling in the face, bad vision, or flashes of light. Your blood tests may also show certain changes that your health-care provider will want to discuss with you.

The women at highest risk for pre-eclampsia are those who have a multiple pregnancy, have had a pre-eclampsia before, or have a medical condition such as hypertension or kidney disease (see the sidebar for other important risk factors). Pre-eclampsia can cause leaky blood vessels in the kidneys. This produces protein in the urine, and high levels of swelling (read about normal swelling on page 90). Extreme complications can include strokes, seizures, liver damage, and blood clotting problems.

All types of high blood pressure are a concern for your baby. High blood pressure can cause poor growth, and may even require early delivery.

Treatment for high blood pressure in pregnancy

Some kinds of high blood pressure during pregnancy may be treated by having the woman rest. If you develop high blood pressure, you may be asked to stop work to allow yourself more rest time at home. Your health-care provider might also prescribe blood pressure medications to keep your blood pressure at a safe level for you and your baby.

Group B Streptococcus (GBS)

At about 36 weeks, you will likely be tested for Group B Streptococcus (GBS) bacteria. This is different from strep throat. However, if you pass these bacteria on to your baby during childbirth, there is a remote chance your baby could become infected too. Babies with GBS infection may have mild to severe problems that may affect their blood, brain, lungs, and spinal cord.

GBS bacteria are usually found in your vagina or rectum. They can infect your bladder, kidneys, or uterus. Infections from GBS are usually not serious for the mother, but can be for the baby. They can be treated easily with antibiotics.

Testing for Group B Streptococcus

The most common way to test a woman for GBS bacteria is to swab her vagina and rectum with a Q-tip. This is then placed in special liquid to see if the bacteria grow. This is called "*doing a culture*." Sometimes your health-care provider may also test for bacteria in your urine.

Treatment for Group B Streptococcus (GBS)

If at 36 weeks you test positive for GBS, you will be offered antibiotics during labour. If you have not been tested for GBS and fall into a high-risk group (see text in sidebar), then you may be treated with antibiotics during labour.

What to expect in the hospital

Obstetrical health care in Canada has changed since your mother gave birth to you, and even more since her mother was "confined" with childbirth. While this may be hard to believe, at one time the process of giving birth was treated as an illness.

YOU MAY BE AT HIGHER RISK TO PASS GROUP B STREPTOCOCCUS (GBS) ON TO YOUR BABY IF YOU:

- *start labour before you reach 37 weeks*
- *reach full term, but your membranes rupture more than 18 hours before your expected time of delivery*
- *have an unexplained mild fever*
- *have already had a baby who had a GBS infection*
- *have (or had) a bladder or kidney infection that was caused by the GBS bacteria*

Childbirth is a normal life experience, not an illness.

FAMILY-CENTRED CARE HOSPITAL CHECKLIST

As you read the list put a check mark beside each statement that is true about your hospital. My hospital:

☐ *Will accept the birth plan I have prepared or has a standard birth plan I can change to suit my needs.*

☐ *Will encourage me to have a labour coach or offers the support of a professional labour coach.*

☐ *Welcomes skin-to-skin contact (kangaroo care) right after birth.*

☐ *Encourages breastfeeding right after birth.*

☐ *Will not separate my baby and me unless it is necessary for medical reasons.*

☐ *Treats birth as a normal and natural process, not an illness.*

☐ *Will try to assign one nurse to me during my labour and delivery (if possible).*

☐ *Accepts my religious beliefs, and wants to do all they can to meet my cultural needs.*

(Continued)

Over the past 20 years or so, doctors, midwives, nurses, and mothers have worked to change the way obstetrics (the delivery of babies) is approached in Canada. Family-centred maternity care has replaced a narrow medical approach. Routine hospital practices were studied to make sure they truly helped women and met their needs. Some standard procedures—such as giving women an enema and an episiotomy—were dropped from routine care. Others—such as birthing rooms—were added.

Modern obstetric units in hospitals have changed to meet and respond to women's needs. Many are warm and home-like. They create a place that welcomes women and their partners—a comforting place that still offers excellent medical care when needed.

Care is usually tailored to the woman's unique needs. That's why women are encouraged to prepare a birth plan that reflects their choices and desires.

Most hospitals in Canada now promote the family-centred approach. It improves the safety of childbirth for the mother and makes the event more enjoyable for all. When hospital maternity care programs include every member of the family, they help families become stronger and healthier. Your partner and your family will be able to offer you more support when they feel needed and included in the childbirth process. Although it is usually best not to have young children present during labour and childbirth, they can welcome the new family member soon after the birth.

Support during labour

The people who surround and support you during labour play an important role. Of course, there will be fewer problems with labour and birth if an experienced health-care professional works closely with you. The ideal for most women is to also have your obstetrician, nurse, or midwife take care of you and your baby after the birth. However, studies show you are more likely to have a normal labour and birth if you have a support person with you—other than a health-care professional. This person might be your partner, family member, friend, or a professional doula.

Rooming in

In family-centred care, most babies "room in." This means they stay in their mother's hospital room and not in the newborn nursery. In most cases, it is healthy and best for mothers and their newborns to stay in the same room from the moment of birth until the time they leave for home.

In the past, having a newborn stay in the nursery was thought to be cleaner and safer than staying in the room with you. In fact, the opposite is true. When an infant stays in the same room as the mother, the mother does most of the care, which reduces risk of infection from other babies and additional handling.

Writing your birth plan

A birth plan is a document that tells your health-care provider and the hospital staff:

- What kind of childbirth you would like.
- How you would like your baby cared for after he is born.

Many hospitals now have a draft birth plan for you to use. You can also use the one provided by the Society of Obstetricians and Gynaecologists of Canada on their website:

www.sogc.org/health/pregnancy-birth-plan_e.asp

FAMILY-CENTRED CARE HOSPITAL CHECKLIST (CONTINUED)

☐ *Allows me to be part of decisions about procedures, labour positions, delivery positions, and pain control.*

☐ *Has flexible visiting hours for close family members.*

If you checked most of these boxes, your hospital offers a family-centred approach to maternity care. If not, then most health-care workers will still try very hard to meet your needs.

BIRTH PLAN

Try not to be too detailed or complex. No one can predict how your labour and birth will progress, so it is important to leave room for change. Remember, the goal of birth is a healthy mother and a healthy baby.

How to write a birth plan

Simple and short is best. It should be less than one page long. Try to be realistic and be aware that your childbirth will include your health-care team, yourself, your partner, the baby, and your family. Your birth plan works best if you write down what you want and what you would prefer if things do not happen as you planned. For example, you may write, "I would prefer not to have an intravenous needle during labour. But if the staff think I need one for a clear medical reason, then I would agree to have one, but only if, and when, it is needed."

When to write a birth plan

Most women write a birth plan after they talk over their childbirth plans with a health-care provider and once they know what their hospital offers in terms of routines and care. It's also a good idea to discuss the plan with your partner and your family if they are going to be involved in some way. However, it is your body, and your family needs to understand that you are the only one who can make some of the more personal decisions (pain control, for example).

Common things included in a birth plan

We have listed some of the common things women include in their birth plans. You do not have to include all of them in your own birth plan. If something is not as important to you, you can leave it out. If you think of something else that is not on this list, feel free to include it.

The labour coach

Studies show that when a woman in labour has the continuous support of someone who cares for her (a labour coach), she will have a more positive experience. The hospital will provide you with a professional labour coach (an obstetrical nurse) who will help you during labour and delivery, and after the baby is born.

Enema

Today's health-care providers do not usually give enemas to women in labour. **An enema** is a liquid put into the rectum to clear out the bowel. However, some women find that having an enema gets rid of pressure in the lower bowel. This is most helpful if they were constipated before labour.

Shaving

Most hospitals no longer shave a woman's pubic area.

Intravenous line (IV)

Unless your pregnancy is high-risk or there is a medical reason, most hospitals will not insert an intravenous line (IV). An IV provides direct and immediate access to your blood stream quickly, in case an emergency happens. Sometimes, an IV is the best way to give you certain medicines—such as antibiotics, or drugs to start labour. Some women benefit from the extra fluids they can get through an IV. It can help prevent dehydration during labour. If you want an epidural (see page 139), you will need to have an IV. Talk to your health-care provider for more information or to decide whether you will use an IV.

Blood tests

If your pregnancy is thought to be low-risk and normal, routine blood tests are not usually done when you first arrive in the labour room. Sometimes, certain blood tests are needed (such as blood sugar tests if you are diabetic) to make sure all is going well.

Inducing labour

If your labour has not started by the end of your 41st week, or if you have other medical problems, your health-care provider may suggest that labour be *induced* (started using medical means). Labour should not be induced without good reason. (Read the section about overdue babies on page 121.)

Augmenting labour

If your labour is moving too slowly, your health-care provider may suggest rupture of membranes or starting an IV with oxytocin. Oxytocin is a hormone that is almost the same as your natural labour hormone. It will cause the contractions to get stronger or become more regular.

Monitoring the baby

Evidence shows that during normal labour, it is best to monitor the baby at regular intervals. This needs to happen in a way that does not limit your movements. If you have special needs, it may be necessary to monitor the baby using continuous fetal monitors, but this should be used only when needed (see page 129).

Movement during labour

Most hospitals today encourage mothers to move about freely during the early stages of labour because studies show that this mild form of exercise helps speed up labour.

Eating and drinking during labour

In the very early stages of labour, eating and drinking small amounts prevents you from getting dehydrated and helps you keep up your strength. However, most women in active labour do not feel like eating. They may want to have small amounts of clear fluids. If some high-risk problems exist, you may not be allowed any food or drink.

Pain relief

There are many different ways to help you cope with the pain of labour and childbirth. These range from special breathing to an epidural block. When your pain is under control, it is easier for you to help with the birth. It's okay to choose natural childbirth (no pain relief), but it's also okay to change your mind if the pain becomes too much for you. You can read more about ways to make labour easier in Chapter Six.

Pushing

At the end of active labour, the urge to push your baby out suddenly becomes strong. The body naturally wants to bear down (push) a few short times during each contraction. Remember to take breaths in and out between pushes. There is proof that this way of pushing gives the baby the most oxygen. Sometimes, hospital staff might ask you to push a different way. You may be encouraged to take a deep breath and hold it, then push one hard, long push with a deep breath at the end. Evidence shows this method may speed up delivery, but it may also lower the baby's oxygen levels over time.

Sometimes, the cervix is not quite ready for the baby to move through. You may be told not to push. If that happens, you will be told what you can do to avoid pushing (such as a knee-to-chest posture or special breathing).

Delivery positions

The best positions for delivery are sitting upright or semi-sitting. These postures seem to lower the time it takes to push a baby out. Lying on your side is also a natural delivery position that has many benefits. Squatting down can be helpful because it improves the angle of the pelvis, giving the baby more room to come out. It also lets gravity do some of the work in helping the baby slide out more quickly. You do not have to worry about having your legs strapped into stirrups. Today's hospitals do not do that.

Episiotomy

There is no evidence to support doing an *episiotomy* for all women (making a cut to widen the opening to the vagina). In fact, there are more benefits to NOT doing this, such as:

• less pain after the baby is born,
• better sexual function later, and
• less relaxation of the pelvic muscles.

In some cases, an episiotomy is necessary to relieve pressure, or to deliver a baby in distress more quickly.

Cutting the umbilical cord

Waiting at least two minutes after the baby is born before cutting the umbilical cord may help your baby get more blood supply. This may be most helpful for premature babies. If your partner wishes to cut the cord, this can also be arranged.

Skin-to-skin contact

Studies show that cuddling and skin-to-skin contact with your baby right after birth helps your baby adjust to life outside the womb and makes breastfeeding easier. This is called kangaroo care.

Religious or cultural beliefs

Feel free to list your needs in this area. You may have customs, beliefs, and certain things you want for yourself, the baby, and your family.

Rooming in

Studies show it is best for you and your new baby to stay and sleep in the same room. Babies who do so are handled mostly by their mothers. Babies in the nursery are handled by many people. Therefore, the risk of infection for a baby is higher in the nursery. By rooming in, you and your baby have a chance to bond with each other.

Caesarean birth

If you know you will be having a Caesarean section (see page 149), you may want to think about what kind of pain relief you want, and if you want your partner to attend. If you were to need an emergency birth, what would your choices be? Include these in your birth plan.

Starting to breastfeed

Evidence shows that the best time to begin breastfeeding is within 30 to 60 minutes after birth, when the baby is most alert. This is also the perfect time to begin bonding with your baby. You can have your baby placed on your belly right after birth, so you both get a good start. This skin-to-skin contact makes it more likely that breastfeeding will be a success. Many babies have the instinct that enables them to know how to breastfeed when they are skin-to-skin.

Feeding schedules

Studies show it is best to breastfeed when your baby seems hungry, and not based on a schedule. This is called feeding on cue. If you watch your baby, you will get to know the cues (or signs) of hunger, such as sucking on the fist, searching with the head for a breast, or crying. Babies should feed at least 8 times during a 24-hour period. You may need to wake your baby up to feed if she is too sleepy to do so.

Just breast milk

Studies show that breastfed babies aged 0–6 months do not need feedings of anything other than breast milk. Water feedings are not necessary.

Asking for help

There are many ways that you can find help for breastfeeding. Sometimes the help will be offered, and sometimes you may have to ask for it. Many communities offer home nursing programs, breastfeeding support through public health clinics, breastfeeding clinics, and professional lactation (breastfeeding) consultants.

Umbilical cord blood banks

After your baby is born and the umbilical cord is cut and clamped, a length of umbilical cord is still linked to the placenta. This cord is filled with a small amount of blood, some of which is tested for the baby's blood type and some other vital levels. The rest of the blood, along with the placenta (once it is expelled), is thrown away as medical waste.

The blood in the umbilical cord contains special cells called *stem cells* which can be used to treat children with cancers or other bone marrow diseases such as leukemia or lymphoma. In other words, these cells could save someone's life.

If you choose to use or donate the umbilical cord blood, you should let your health-care providers know. Include this in your birth plan. Umbilical cord blood must be taken after birth, but before the placenta is delivered. This blood can be banked for use in the near future, but there is no proof that it can be stored for long periods and still be used to treat cancer or disease. Cord blood banks require that you go through a screening process. You will need to contact your local bank before you reach 34 weeks to complete the screening process.

In Canada, there are a limited number of public umbilical cord banks who store blood for the public good.

The following websites provide more information on umbilical cord blood banking:

- *The Society of Obstetricians and Gynaecologists of Canada: www.sogc.org*
- *The Alberta Cord Blood Bank: www.acbb.ca*
- *Hema-Quebec: www.hema-quebec.qc.ca*

Feeding your baby

Over the past 20 years, breastfeeding has been studied a great deal. Research shows that it offers many clear benefits for both the mother and the child. Based on this scientific evidence, the Society of Obstetricians and Gynaecologists of Canada (SOGC), the Canadian Paediatric Society (CPS), the World Health Organization (WHO), and the United Nation's Children's Fund (UNICEF) agree that the best food source for the first six months of life is breast milk. After six months of only breastfeeding, you can begin to give the baby other foods. It is good to continue breastfeeding until your child is two years old or even older.

Breastfeeding—the natural and healthy way to feed your baby

Women have always breastfed their children. Breastfeeding is still the healthiest and most natural way to feed your baby. Today, 85% of Canadian mothers will breastfeed.

Breast milk, including the first milk that your breasts produce (colostrum), contains antibodies that complete your baby's immune system and help fight disease. A strong immune system lowers the chance of your baby getting infections such as colds, ear infections, stomach flu, kidney infections, pneumonia, and meningitis. Breastfed babies also have a lower chance of getting certain bowel problems such as celiac disease or Crohn's disease. Breast milk even lowers the chances of developing appendicitis, asthma, allergies, and eczema.

Breast milk is more easily absorbed and quicker to digest than formula. That's why breastfed babies tend to have fewer problems with constipation and stomach upset. Babies are hardly ever allergic to breast milk, but they can have mild to severe allergic reactions to formula. Breast milk also contains active proteins that support the development of your baby's gut, nerves, and disease-fighting cells.

BREASTFEEDING STARTS WITH COLOSTRUM

Most babies are ready to breastfeed within the first hour after they are born. Until your milk volume increases (usually two to four days after the birth), your breasts will produce a yellow, milk-like substance called colostrum. This colostrum has antibodies, omega-3 fatty acids, and the perfect balance of nutrients, minerals, vitamins, and trace elements for your baby.

Your baby will be born with extra water and fat to use until the amount of milk in your body rises. In the meantime, the colostrum feedings are perfect for baby and all she needs.

Most babies lose weight after birth because they use up the fat and water stored in their bodies. This weight loss should not be more than 7% of their birth weight.

It is best to breastfeed your newborn whenever he shows signs of being hungry (sucking on his fist, smacking his lips, trying to suck on anything near him). Babies should not be given water.

Breastfeeding is also very good for you, the mother. It triggers the release of certain hormones that help your uterus return to its normal size. Breastfeeding also helps protect you from cancer of the breast, ovaries, and uterus. Breastfeeding allows you and your baby to feel closeness and a special bond. Finally, breastfeeding is free and needs no time to prepare. Formula feeding could cost $1,500 or more during the first year.

Talk to other women and to organizations such as the La Leche League Canada Breastfeeding Referral Service (1-800-665-4324) or your local public health nurse to learn more. In some places, breastfeeding clinics and private breastfeeding experts, called lactation consultants, are also available to help you.

Sometimes, some women choose not to breastfeed. If you decide not to breastfeed (see page 193 for more information), your health-care providers will respect your choice and support you.

Breastfeeding myths—true and false:

1. Breastfeeding is easy, natural, and based on human instinct.

   True. Once you and your baby have started and then developed your own routine, breastfeeding is easy and the most natural way to feed a baby. Like many new things you are learning to do with your new baby, it can take time to get it right. Be patient with yourself. Ask for help. Stay with your decision—it's worth it.

2. I shouldn't start breastfeeding because I'm not sure I can continue for more than two or three months.

   False. It is worthwhile for your baby to be breastfed for any amount of time, even if it's just for a few days. This way, your baby will get the advantages of your milk and you will be able to keep your options open. So, even if you do not know how long you will be able to breastfeed, it's worth starting.

3. Mothers who breastfeed are "tied" to their babies.

True. But then, all new mothers are "tied" to their babies! Breastfeeding or not, your newborn will need frequent feedings and care. Yes, breastfeeding mothers do need to stay close to their babies, which is natural. You will feel good knowing that you are there to breastfeed and comfort your baby. Unlike formula, no additional time or special preparations are required for breastfeeding. In the early months, take the baby with you. You will likely find breastfeeding offers you both convenience and flexibility. Some new mothers feel lonely and miss the regular contact with other adults. Make sure you keep in touch with friends, or make new ones.

4. Every woman can produce enough milk to feed her baby.

True. Breastfeeding your baby promotes your body's milk supply so you can meet your baby's exact demands. Sometimes a mother thinks she is not producing enough milk. In most cases, these doubts can be addressed by talking to a person trained in breastfeeding. If you think you are not producing enough milk, talk to your health-care provider or find a program in your community that supports breastfeeding mothers. In most cases, the problem can be solved or explained. Sometimes, a mother can give her baby more of her own milk (by pumping milk from her breasts). In rare cases, a woman may need to offer more than breast milk (formula) until the problem is solved.

5. Babies must suck in a different way from a bottle than from a breast.

True. Babies who are bottle-fed need to learn a different type of sucking than breastfed babies. It is true that babies may become confused by the difference between your nipple and the nipple of a bottle.

6. Breastfeeding will change the way my breasts look.

True. In the first few weeks of breastfeeding, expect your breasts to increase in size. Once you stop, your breasts may be a different shape than they were before pregnancy. This is due to pregnancy hormones and age—not breastfeeding.

7. If I breastfeed, I should not bottle feed at all.

It depends. At the start, you are more likely to have success with breastfeeding if you do not give your baby a bottle at all. This way your baby will not get confused by the different nipples. As well, the way your body produces milk will match your baby's demand. Once your milk supply and the baby's technique are well set (at least six weeks after birth), you can begin to give the baby a bottle, sometimes. The best thing to put in that bottle is breast milk that you have pumped (expressed). Please be aware that giving your baby a bottle at any time raises the chance that the baby will be weaned (end of breastfeeding) early.

8. Children should be weaned at six months of age.

False. Breast milk is the best milk for babies and toddlers. The World Health Organization (WHO) recommends only breastfeeding for the first six months of life, and continued breastfeeding for up to two years and beyond. If breastfeeding is working well for you, there is no reason to quit before your child does so on his or her own.

9. Some mothers should not breastfeed.

True, but this is very rare. In some cases, a health-care provider may advise a woman not to breastfeed. For example, a woman may need to take medicines that could harm the child if she breastfeeds. Talk to your health-care provider about breastfeeding and any medicines that you take.

10. Women with breast implants cannot breastfeed.

False. Many women with implants can breastfeed.

11. Blue or watery milk has no nutritional value.

False. The way breast milk looks may change as the breast gets softer during a feed. As the breast gets softer, the fat content of the milk rises. All breast milk has nutritional value for your baby.

12. The small amount of colostrum is enough for your baby in the first few days.

    True. Colostrum provides both water and sugar, as well as protein, minerals and important antibodies that your baby cannot get from anything but breast milk.

13. Breastfed babies should be given a soother (pacifier) to help them learn to suck.

    False. A soother may teach your baby poor sucking technique. It may hide the baby's hunger signs from you and it can spread disease. See Chapter Eight for more details on this.

14. It is best to breastfeed a baby whenever she seems hungry.

    True. Breastfeeding your baby on cue makes for a more satisfied baby and success with breastfeeding. Most babies feed at least 8 times during a 24-hour period.

15. Both breastfed and bottle-fed babies need to have water.

    False. Breast milk contains enough water to meet your baby's needs. Water has no nutritional value, and feeding your baby water can make the baby less hungry at feeding time.

16. If I am going to breastfeed, I will have to eat properly.

    True. But you have to eat properly to meet your own needs anyway! It is always wise, whether breastfeeding or not, to practice good nutrition. Eating well helps you recover from the baby's birth and helps your body heal.

17. I have to wean my baby before I go back to work.

    False. Mothers who return to work have a number of choices. Some mothers breastfeed when they are at home and pump (or express) their milk while at work, for the baby to have the next day. Other mothers breastfeed when they are at home and use frozen breast milk or formula when they are away.

My pregnancy journal
24 to 32 weeks

During your exam, your health-care provider will weigh and measure you and your baby. As with your last visit, your health-care provider will discuss the signs of preterm labour with you and how well you are reducing the risks. Are you eating well and getting regular exercise? Are you protecting your baby from cigarette smoke and alcohol? Is your work stressful or does it make you very tired? Do you get enough rest?

If you have had any tests or a screening ultrasound since your last visit, your health-care provider will review the results with you.

Together, you will also review your plans for childbirth and what you can expect. Talking about these things, combined with the reading you are doing, will help you get a clear picture of the choices you have for birthing your baby. You will start to think about how you want to proceed, based on what you think is best for you, your baby, and your partner.

KEEPING TRACK OF MY PROGRESS

Date:

Week of pregnancy:

Blood pressure:

Weight:

Fetal heart rate:

THINGS TO DISCUSS WITH MY HEALTH-CARE PROVIDER:

Questions about breastfeeding:

Questions about my birth plan:

Weight gain/nutrition:

Other concerns:

My pregnancy journal
32 to 36 weeks

You will have prenatal visits every two to three weeks. Both you and your baby will be weighed and measured and your health-care provider will continue to look for any signs of preterm labour. Your baby's health and growth will be the focus of these visits.

You and your health-care provider will review your birth plan at this visit (see page 101) and talk about any concerns you may have about childbirth.

Eating well is still very important, because your baby is growing quickly.

KEEPING TRACK OF MY PROGRESS

Date:

Week of pregnancy:

Blood pressure:

Weight:

Fetal heart rate:

THINGS TO DISCUSS WITH MY HEALTH-CARE PROVIDER:

Questions about breastfeeding:

Questions about my birth plan:

Weight gain/nutrition:

Other concerns:

115

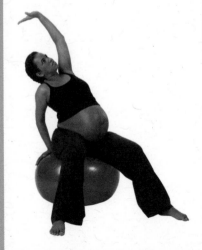

_____
_____
_____
_____
_____
_____
_____
_____
_____
_____
_____
_____
_____
_____
_____
_____
_____
_____
_____
_____
_____

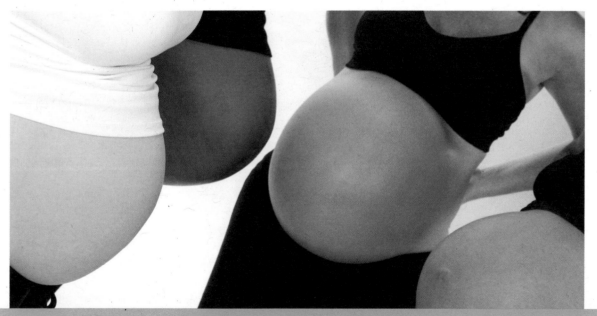

Chapter Five

Getting ready to give birth

IMPORTANT THINGS TO THINK
ABOUT BEFORE LABOUR BEGINS:

- *How easy will it be to reach your labour support partner when you go into labour?*

- *Do you have an alternate person you can contact?*

- *How do you plan to get to the hospital?*

- *Who will drive you there? You should not drive yourself to the hospital. You will need to focus on yourself. You may not be able to drive safely when you are in labour.*

- *If you are using your own car, can you depend on it? Make a back-up plan, just in case there is trouble with the car.*

- *If you plan to take a taxi, make sure you have taxi money. Contact social services if you need funds to help you get to the hospital.*

- *How far are you from the hospital? It is best to drive the distance and use a clock to record how long it takes to make the journey.*

(Continued)

Introduction

Well, if you are getting a little tired of carrying your baby, how do you think your baby is feeling? So, just as pilots go through a final checklist before take-off, welcome to your final checklist before childbirth. Who's going to run the video camera? What about your toothbrush? Parking? Oh, and do you think your baby might be getting ready in her own way?

We'll talk about common "late discomforts" that you may be feeling. And now is the time to discuss overdue babies and some of the signs and concerns.

Be aware that the end of your pregnancy is near and that you are very close to holding the newest member of your family.

Your changing body

Your pelvic bones have loosened and may ache, especially at the back. You may notice your breasts leaking some colostrum, leaving a thin crust on your nipples (although many women do not produce colostrum before the baby is born). Your breasts may feel full and heavy. You will need a good support bra for the months to come, especially if you breastfeed. Your belly may become so stretched that your navel pushes out. Near the end of your pregnancy, you may notice that the colour of your skin (pigmentation) looks browner and becomes stronger near the end of pregnancy.

Your uterus will begin "practice contractions" (also called "Braxton Hicks contractions") that may or may not be painless. They will be irregular. Because the uterus is putting a lot of pressure on the blood vessels in your pelvis, you may notice more swelling in your feet and ankles. But if your hands and face swell, it may be the sign of a more serious problem, such as gestational hypertension (see page 97). If this happens, contact your health-care provider.

Near the end of pregnancy, most babies will settle into the head down, or "engaged" position. The event is also known as "when the baby drops" or "lightening." For some women, this does not happen until just before labour starts, which is normal.

When your baby settles into your pelvis, the head will rest on top of your cervix. You will feel different and it will appear that you are carrying the baby much lower than you were before. The good news is that after the baby drops, some of the pressure on your ribs will be lifted. Breathing will be easier. Sometimes, the low and heavy weight that happens now can add to a feeling of muscle strain and backache.

Your baby at full term

Your full-term baby is plump and rounded and measures 46–51 cm (18–20 inches) in length, and weighs between 3 and 4 kilograms (6-1/2 to 9 pounds).

The baby's eyes are open when awake, and closed when sleeping. Her lungs are now producing a substance called surfactant that will help her take the first breath. A full-term baby's immune system is still not fully developed. To solve this problem, your placenta will continue to provide antibodies to the baby before birth. Your breast milk (colostrum) will do the same after birth. The placenta now measures about 20 cm (8–10 inches) across and is about 2.5 cm (1 inch) thick.

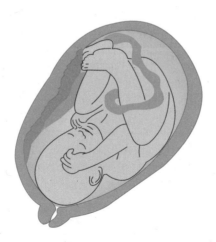

▶ *Your baby at full term*

IMPORTANT THINGS TO THINK ABOUT BEFORE LABOUR BEGINS: (CONTINUED)

• *How will this timing change if road conditions are bad, there are detours, or the city is building or repairing roads? What if the weather is bad, or if you must travel during rush hour traffic? Plan different routes to avoid any problems you can think of.*

• *Where are you supposed to park the car? Do you need to pre-register at the hospital or can you just arrive?*

• *Who will take care of your children at home?*

• *Do you need someone to feed your pets while you are in the hospital?*

• *Create your "Labour action list and Contact list" for the Big Day (see pages 217 and 218).*

PACKING YOUR SUITCASE

You are going on a trip, so you need to pack a suitcase a few weeks before your due date, in case the baby arrives early. Once labour begins, you may not have time to pack everything you want to take with you.

PACKING CHECKLIST FOR YOU:

☐ *this book, pen, and paper*
☐ *copy of your birth plan*
☐ *housecoat, nightgown, and slippers*
☐ *loose-fitting clothing to go home in*
☐ *extra pair of socks*
☐ *bra (breastfeeding or good support bra)*
☐ *underwear*
☐ *sanitary napkins*
☐ *toothbrush and toothpaste*
☐ *hairbrush, comb*
☐ *camera and batteries*
☐ *coins for phones and vending machines*
☐ *labour support items, such as massage oil for back rubs*

PACKING CHECKLIST FOR YOUR BABY:

☐ *clothing to go home in*
☐ *diaper(s)*
☐ *receiving blanket*
☐ *warmer blanket*
☐ *hat*
☐ *car seat*

Common discomforts in late pregnancy

Leg, calf, and foot cramps

Many women feel these kinds of cramps during the last three months of pregnancy, mostly at night. They are sudden cramps in the thighs, legs, calves, or feet. When you get a cramp, try this:

• In spite of the pain, point your toes up, toward your knee. This will help to stretch the muscle.
• Keep your foot in this flexed position while you slowly and carefully make circles with your lower leg.
• Then, massage the cramped muscle to improve the blood supply to that part of your body.

Problems sleeping

Sleeping problems are common throughout pregnancy, but most common in the final trimester. Your enlarged belly makes it hard to find a comfortable position, and the added trips to the bathroom at night do not help either. Try using two or three large pillows to support your legs, belly, and back (but do not lie flat on your back). Ask your partner for a back massage to help you drift off to sleep. It may help to take a warm bath before going to bed. Try keeping the bedroom temperature cool. Do not take sleeping pills unless your health-care provider approves them.

Discharge from your vagina

Discharge from your vagina usually increases during pregnancy. During your last trimester, it can become even more plentiful. The discharge should not be:

• white or bloody (unless your cervix has begun to open and your mucus plug is released, which may happen a few days before labour starts)
• watery (this could be amniotic fluid)
• foul-smelling (this may mean you have an infection)

You should not feel any pain, itching, or soreness in your vaginal area. Contact your health-care provider right away if you have any of these signs or you think there might be a problem.

Pre-labour contractions

Pre-labour contractions (you may also hear them called Braxton Hicks contractions) are usually light and painless, and do not occur in any regular pattern. They're normal and are thought to be the muscles of your uterus preparing for labour. Many women do not even notice when they happen. They are different from the contractions that come with labour—which begin slowly, and then become more frequent, stronger and regular in occurrence. Refer to the sidebar for further discussion about "true labour" and "false labour." But, if you are concerned that you may be in labour, seek an assessment by a health-care provider.

Overdue babies

About 10% of women will not give birth to their babies by the end of their 41st week, or within one week after their due date. When a pregnancy goes beyond the 42nd week, it is called *post-term* and the baby is said to be *overdue*. To be sure your pregnancy is truly post-term, your baby's due date must be accurate. Your due date will have been calculated early in your pregnancy using the date of your last menstrual period and the results of the earliest ultrasound of your pregnancy. Trying to calculate due dates late in pregnancy using uncertain menstrual dates or late ultrasounds is not reliable.

An aging placenta

A small number of overdue babies will develop health problems. We do not know why a few overdue babies have these problems, but it may be because of an aging placenta. As it gets older, the placenta begins to lose its ability to do its job. When this happens, it may mean that fewer

---

TRUE LABOUR VS. FALSE LABOUR

If you do not know if your labour is true or false, it's helpful to time the contractions and note how strong and regular they are. Write down how many minutes apart they are, from the start of one contraction until the start of the next, and note how long each one lasts. If possible, keep a record for one hour.

1. HOW STRONG ARE THE CONTRACTIONS?

TRUE LABOUR
- *The contractions will gradually get stronger over time.*
- *You will be able to feel your uterus becoming firmer.*

FALSE LABOUR
- *The contractions do not gradually get stronger over time.*
- *They may weaken at times and even go away for a while.*

(Continued)

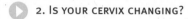

True labour vs. false labour (continued)

▶ **2. Is your cervix changing?**

True labour

- *Your cervix begins to change as it softens, shortens, and opens.*

- *If the cervix opens to 3 or 4 cm with regular contractions, this is a sign of active labour.*

False labour

- *There is no change in your cervix.*

- *It does not soften, shorten, thin out, or open up.*

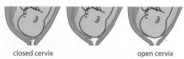

closed cervix   open cervix

▶ **3. How regular are the contractions?**

True labour

- *The contractions usually become quite regular. You can predict them.*

- *In true labour, contractions last 30 to 70 seconds and happen about five minutes apart (or less).*

False labour

- *The contractions are not regular and never really settle down into a pattern.*

nutrients and less blood and oxygen reach your baby. In some cases, this can cause stress for your baby and slow his growth.

Making sure your overdue baby is safe

If your baby is still not born after your 41st week, or within a week after your due date, you and your health-care provider will discuss whether or not to induce labour (see Chapter Six for many more details). To help you decide whether this is right for you, you will need to keep close track of what the baby is doing, as when you counted the baby's movements (see page 96). You may also need to have a test that measures the fetal heart rate (non-stress testing), as well as an ultrasound.

My pregnancy journal
36 to 42 weeks

You will have prenatal exams every week during the last four to six weeks of your pregnancy. At each visit, your health-care provider will examine both you and your baby closely. The goal is to make sure that you are both making good progress and that your body is getting ready for the big event: childbirth.

CHAPTER SIX

Your time is here

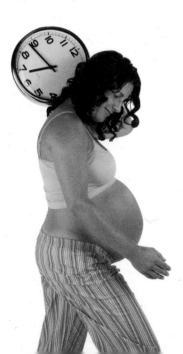

IF YOU ARE EXPECTING TWINS OR MULTIPLES

With twins or multiples, your labour experience may be slightly different from what is described in this chapter. You should already have discussed what to expect with your health-care provider or a specialist. This chapter will help you learn the basics of labour and birth.

Introduction

You have arrived at the moment everyone has been waiting for. In this chapter, we'll discuss the signs of labour, followed by the four stages of labour. We'll talk about your "water breaking," breathing, positions, pain relief, and assisted birth techniques. We even have a section on bonding.

As usual, we'll also talk about possible risks and problems. One of our goals has been to reduce the number of surprises for you. And, because it happens, we'll also discuss the worst-case scenario.

So, after months of waiting (and maybe when you least expect it), you'll begin to feel the start of labour. Like most women, you may feel surprised, excited, and even a little afraid. But yours is the major role in the final act of this nine-month miracle—the growth of a fertilized egg that was smaller than the dot over the "i" in the word "life" into a living, breathing human being. You are about to experience the joy of bringing a new life into your family.

When labour begins

No one can truly predict when your labour will begin. There is no single thing that prompts labour, although we think hormones play an important role. So, this section will prepare you for the signs of labour and help you be ready to respond.

Signs of labour

Some women know they are in labour right away. Others may not be so sure. Sometimes, it is even hard for the experts to know. If you are in doubt, you should go to the hospital.

Show: During your pregnancy, a mucus plug forms at the opening of your cervix. When your cervix begins to open (or dilate), this plug is released.

You may notice a thick discharge from your vagina. This is called "show." It may have some blood in it. Or it may appear clear or pinkish. This may happen many days before labour starts, so you will need to wait for further signs that labour has begun.

Ruptured membrane: You may have heard the expression that your "water will break." The medical term is ruptured membrane. Both refer to the same thing: when the sac of amniotic fluid around your baby begins leaking or breaks open fully. This can happen many hours before labour begins, or at any time during labour. Go to the hospital if this happens.

Contractions: Labour often begins with contractions of the uterus, when your uterus gets tight and then relaxes. These contractions happen so that your cervix will open and help move the baby down the birth canal. (See pages 121 and 122 to help you tell the difference between true and false labour.)

Labour contractions are painful and regular, and usually last somewhere between 30 and 70 seconds.

The importance of your labour coach

You will feel more comfortable during labour if you see a familiar face. You can choose anyone you wish to be your labour coach, such as your partner, the baby's father, a friend, a family member, and (or) a doula (a trained labour coach). Coaches can offer you the emotional support you need, rub your aching back if it helps, remind you of the special breathing routines you learned in prenatal classes, and hold your hand when you need it most. Some hospitals have volunteers to help women in labour.

I'M HAVING CONTRACTIONS—IS THIS LABOUR?

A number of factors will help you determine if you're in labour—when in doubt, you should contact, or see, a health-care provider.

Once you experience contractions, the key factors for you to consider (which you should also write down) are:

- *Frequency of contractions—Time and record your contractions, from the start of the contraction to the end, as well as how often they occur, e.g., first contractions last 30 seconds and occur 10 minutes apart.*

- *Strength of contractions—How strong are they? Can you feel your uterus actually becoming "hard," and are the contractions causing discomfort, or pain (usually in the lower abdomen, or back)?*

- *Duration—For how long have you been having the contractions, i.e., have you been having them for a couple of hours, all afternoon, or . . . ?*

Helping your labour coach prepare

Labour coaches need to prepare, especially if this is their first birth. They may wonder how they will help during labour. Some may worry about feeling nervous or queasy and not being able to offer enough support.

Here are a few suggestions for your labour coach:

"Hello, Labour Coach. You have a tough job to do. If you are feeling nervous, that is normal, especially if this is your first birth. You want to do all you can to help and protect the mother, and you share her concern for the health of the baby. (If you are the father, it's your baby, too!)

You may feel that you should be 'doing something.' Sometimes, you may feel that these efforts are 'making a difference,' while at other times you may feel that you are somewhat helpless. If all these things describe you, you are normal.

Before labour begins, encourage your partner to rest often and to take care of herself. If you live together, do her share of the cleaning, laundry, and cooking.

If you helped to prepare the birth plan, you know what type of birth you both want. She may need you to be her voice to the hospital staff during her labour.

It will help if you remain as calm as possible. Offer words of praise and encouragement. Help her relax as much as possible between contractions. When you help with special breathing, allow her to follow her own rhythm. Sometimes, her body will tell her which rhythm is best and it may not always be the pattern you learned and practised together.

If she seems to be losing control of her contractions, stay close, talk her quietly through the contraction, keep eye contact, and try to get her back on track for the next one.

Be flexible about her birth plan and do not feel upset if things do not go exactly the way she (and you) planned. Listen carefully to her wishes—they may change. Also listen to the staff—they have done this many times.

Remember to take care of yourself too during this long and stressful process. Take time to eat, drink, and rest."

Your labour and delivery team

In most cases, hospital deliveries begin with meeting your obstetrical nurse when you arrive. Most labour and delivery professionals are registered nurses, but some may have training as midwives. If possible, the same nurse will stay with you during your labour and delivery. Licensed midwives also care for women during pregnancy, labour, and delivery.

Studies show that you will benefit from having a nurse or midwife who is focused on your care. These partners want to help you master techniques to make your labour easier. They are also very experienced, and know when the birth process is going well and when it is not.

The stages of labour

There are four stages of labour:

- Stage 1 begins with the first contractions, when they become regular. It ends when your cervix is fully open (dilated) at 10 centimetres.
- Stage 2 begins when your cervix is fully open (dilated) and ends when your baby is born.
- Stage 3 begins after the baby is born and ends when the placenta is delivered.
- Stage 4 is the immediate time after the birth, during which the mother's condition is stabilized following the delivery—any complications for the mother are addressed at this time.

GO TO THE HOSPITAL WHEN:

- *Your water breaks in a gush, or is leaking steadily.*
- *Your contractions are regular and five minutes apart (and the hospital is less than 30 minutes away).*
- *Your contractions are regular and 10 minutes apart (and the hospital is more than 30 minutes away).*

If you are not sure what to do or how to measure your contractions, call the labour and delivery unit at your hospital.

MONITORING YOUR BABY DURING LABOUR

In a routine pregnancy, the best way to check on a baby's well-being during labour is to listen to its heart through the mother's belly. A nurse or midwife will check the fetal heart rate (FHR) often and regularly by using a stethoscope or a hand-held Doppler (a machine that picks up the sounds of your baby's heart).

(Continued)

During labour, the FHR will be checked:

- *for a full minute after a contraction or about two to four times each hour during the first stage of labour*
- *every five minutes, when you begin the second stage of labour and start pushing*

If your pregnancy or labour is considered high risk, or if a problem arises during labour, your health team may need to use some form of electronic fetal monitoring (EFM) to know how your baby is doing, especially during the contractions. This type of monitor is often used if:

- *your baby's heart rate is too slow or too fast*
- *the baby has had a bowel movement known as **meconium** (the first stool that a baby passes while still in the uterus)*

EFM is very common, but should only be used if there are concerns about the baby's heart rate. It limits a mother's ability to walk around or move freely during labour. Two kinds of EFMs measure and record a baby's heartbeat and the length and strength of the mother's contractions.

(Continued)

The average time for labour is 12 to 14 hours for a first childbirth, and other deliveries are usually shorter. Keep in mind that these are just averages, and that every labour is different. No one can predict what your labour will be like or how long it will last.

Early in pregnancy, your cervix is a thick-walled canal about 2.5 cm (one inch) long. It is closed. During the last few weeks of your pregnancy, hormones will make your cervix soften. This is called the ***ripening*** of the cervix. Once labour begins, contractions make the ripened cervix ***dilate*** (open up) and ***efface*** (thin out). At the end of the first stage of labour, your cervix will be open 10 centimetres (four inches) and the sides will be very thin. At this point, your uterus, cervix, and vagina will shape themselves into one long birth canal for the baby to pass through.

The first stage of labour

The first stage of labour usually lasts the longest. It is divided into three parts: early, active, and transition.

Early (or latent) stage: 0–3 cm

In this early stage, it may be hard to know for sure if you are in labour. Tracking the strength and regularity of your contractions and paying close attention for any changes to your cervix will help you and your health-care provider be certain (see pages 121 to 122). If you go to the hospital during this stage, you will be assessed and then either observed for a few hours or told to go home until your labour truly begins.

During this "latent" or early part of labour, drink fluids and try a warm bath or a shower. Sometimes, if you have been having irregular contractions and you are tired, you may be offered some pain medicine to help you rest and regain your strength for when real labour begins.

Active stage: 3–8 cm

You will notice that your contractions have become much stronger. They last about 45 seconds and occur about every 3 to 5 minutes. As the contractions progress, your cervix will continue to thin and open. At the end of this stage, your cervix should have opened to eight centimetres. You may begin to feel quite tired and anxious. Now is a good time to relax as much as you can between contractions. You may have some back pain because of where the baby's head is sitting in your pelvis.

Transition stage: 8–10 cm

You are almost at the end of stage 1 now. Your contractions may be every two to three minutes and will usually last about 60 to 90 seconds. This helps your cervix to dilate fully to 10 centimetres. In many women, labour actually slows down during the transition stage and it may take longer to dilate the final two centimetres. While your cervix dilates these last couple of centimetres, the baby's head should be moving down slowly into the pelvis.

Medication-free ways to make labour easier

Labour tends to be easier if you are relaxed and feel confident. Many of the techniques that you and your support team will use to make labour easier help you relax and remain in control of your body and mind.

You and your labour coach will have learned and practised many different techniques in the weeks and months before labour began. Remember, a technique that works for other women may not work for you. That's why it's good to have as many techniques as possible at your disposal.

MONITORING YOUR BABY DURING LABOUR (CONTINUED)

Sometimes it is necessary to take a sample of blood from the baby's scalp (fetal scalp sampling) to check blood oxygen and pH levels.

External Monitor	Internal Monitor
• The mother wears a belt around her belly.	• A small electrode attached to a monitor is inserted through the mother's vagina.
• The belt has wires that are attached to the monitor.	• A scalp clip is attached to a part of the baby that can be reached through the open cervix (usually the top of the head).

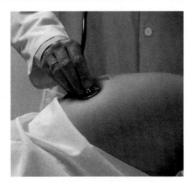

Slow progress in labour is common. How long it should take depends on how many babies you have had. If this is your first childbirth, the time from the start of active labour to childbirth (delivery) averages about 12 to 14 hours. You may be given **oxytocin,** *a synthetic hormone, to make your contractions more effective. This often happens when dilation is slow and your contractions are not frequent or strong enough. Studies have shown that using oxytocin to help with a slow labour can help in two ways:*

- *It prevents labour from going on for too long (exhausting the mother and putting stress on the baby).*

- *It reduces the need for a Caesarean delivery.*

Special breathing

The way you breathe during labour may help make your job easier and give you a sense of control over your body and mind. Sometimes you will just follow your body's lead, and breathe in the way that feels right for you. You may also find some of the following techniques helpful. These three are suited to the three types of early labour.

Slow breathing

Slow, deep breathing works best in the early stage of labour because it shifts your focus away from the contractions. Begin by taking a deep breath through your nose or mouth. Then, purse your lips as if you are blowing up a balloon and very slowly blow the air out. For many women, the rate and rhythm of this kind of breathing comes naturally, but a handy rule is to breathe in for three or four counts, and then out for three or four counts. Many women in labour find that this type of slow breathing helps them all the way through their entire labour.

Light/quick breathing

This type of breathing works best during the active part of labour, when the contractions are coming more often and are getting quite strong. When a contraction begins, start by breathing slowly in and out. As the contraction gets stronger, shorten your breaths. At the peak of the contraction (the strongest point), breathe lightly in and quickly out, making a puffing sound almost like a dog panting. When the contraction starts to ease off, slow your breathing down again and then take a deep, cleansing breath.

Transition breathing (pant-pant-blow)

During the transition stage of labour—when the labour is most intense and you find it hard to breathe slowly—this kind of breathing can help you resist the urge to push against a cervix that is not fully dilated. It is often called "pant-pant-blow breathing" and is done by taking a deep breath in, then exhaling two short pants, followed by a longer blow to empty your lungs.

COPING WITH EARLY LABOUR

YOU CAN:

- *Take a warm bath or a shower.*
- *Walk with your labour coach or watch a movie.*
- *Use relaxation techniques.*
- *Breathe slowly and deeply through contractions.*
- *Keep your energy levels up by eating and drinking lightly.*

YOUR LABOUR COACH CAN:

- *Have the car ready and filled with gas.*
- *Put your bags into the car.*
- *Help you relax by offering you a back or foot massage.*
- *If necessary, let people know labour has started.*
- *Encourage you to walk, rest, eat, and drink.*
- *Time your contractions from the start of one to the start of the next.*
- *Be calm and reassuring.*
- *Prepare a light meal for you; offer you plenty of fluids.*

COPING WITH ACTIVE LABOUR

YOU CAN:

- Relax; go with the flow of contractions.

- Use light/quick breathing or a slow relaxed breathing.

- Change positions often, but do not lie on your back. Moving will speed up labour.

- Expect your contractions to get much stronger after your water breaks.

- Ask for pain relief if you need it.

- Use visualization to help you to focus.

- Take a warm bath or a shower.

- Use a birthing ball to put counter-pressure on your perineum and to help open up your pelvis.

- Ask for help; make your needs known.

YOUR LABOUR COACH CAN:

- Massage tense muscles.

- Stay with you.

- Help with your breathing, letting your rhythm dictate the best breathing pattern for you.

- Encourage and help you to change positions often. Use pillows for support. Walk with you. Help you to sit up if that's what you want to do.

- Apply firm counter-pressure to your back during contractions. Give back massages between contractions.

- Be your voice with the staff.

- Let you focus on your labour.

- Encourage you and tell you how far you have come. Help you get through contractions one at a time and prepare for the next one.

- Support your choices. Never criticize. Make the room as peaceful as possible. Be calm and reassuring.

COPING WITH THE TRANSITION TO SECOND-STAGE LABOUR

YOU CAN:

- Move around as much as you need to get comfortable.

- Try the "pant-pant-blow" breathing to help resist the urge to push if your cervix is not dilated to 10 centimetres.

- Get through your contractions one at a time.

- Take a shower or tub bath if possible.

- Visualize your body opening up like a flower to let your baby move out.

- Use a cool cloth to wash your hands and face.

- Change your gown.

- Suck ice chips or sip water to keep your mouth moist.

- Tell your labour coach or nurse if you have the urge to push.

YOUR LABOUR COACH CAN:

- Support your choice of position.

- Help with breathing. Maintain eye contact so that you feel linked to someone and more in control.

- Remind you that labour is almost over and the baby is nearly out. Be calm and offer positive support.

- Rub tense muscles if you want, especially around the lower back where the baby's head may be applying pressure.

- Help you with visualization and relaxation.

- Stroke your face, hair, or other parts of your body if you find that helps.

- Offer ice chips; apply a cool cloth to your brow.

- Help you to do transition breathing (pant-pant-blow) to avoid pushing until the nurse comes.

Body positions

Your body position can make labour easier. You should feel free to labour in any position that makes the process easier and to change positions as often as you want. Use pillows to prop up your legs, arms, and belly. It is not good to lie flat on your back during labour because the weight of the uterus may squeeze a large blood vessel against your spine, slowing the blood supply to the baby.

Sitting upright

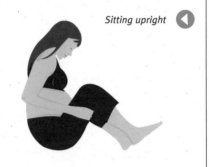

Sitting upright

Sitting up straight (or leaning back slightly) is the most common and best birth position. Studies show that this position may help your uterus to contract and, therefore, may shorten the second stage of labour. As well, the sitting position seems to help the baby move down the birth canal. Further studies show that babies born to mothers who were sitting upright during delivery had better oxygen levels in their blood. Mothers said they liked this position because it was easier to see their baby and they were able to bond with the baby once it was born. Most hospitals have birthing beds that make this sitting position easier.

Lying on your side

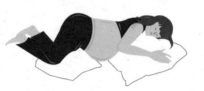

Lying on your side

You may find yourself lying on your side at one time or another during labour but you may not have thought of your baby being born when you are in this position. Some women feel more comfortable labouring on their side. If you have certain heart conditions, hip joint problems, or varicose veins in your legs, this position may help your doctor or midwife deliver your baby safely. If you choose this position, your labour coach will need to support your upper leg during the birth.

Squatting—delivery only

The squatting position has two benefits. First, it makes bearing down (pushing) easier because gravity helps the uterus fall forward. This helps your baby move down the birth canal. Second, studies show that squatting helps widen the pelvis, giving the baby more room to move down and out. North American women sometimes find this position uncomfortable because they are not used to it. Some hospitals provide birthing bars on their birthing beds to help women who want to use this position.

Kneeling on all fours (can be used for delivery, or sometimes late in the first stage)

This position works well for some women, although very few studies have looked at how well it works. Some experts believe it may help a baby turn around into the proper position for delivery if it has not done so on its own. Many women rock back and forth on all fours during contractions to help reduce their backache. This may be a useful position to try.

Hydrotherapy

Hydrotherapy involves the use of water during the first stage of labour as a pain and stress reliever.

Many women in labour find comfort in showers, whirlpool baths, and tub baths. Although hydrotherapy does not appear to shorten labour, when you feel less stressed, your body produces more "feel good" hormones called endorphins. As well, lower stress levels during labour will allow the levels of the hormone oxytocin to rise. This helps to make contractions stronger and more regular.

Before you begin water therapy, it is best to get help from your nurse, midwife, or other support person. Water that is too hot can open (dilate) the blood vessels close to your skin and make your blood pressure drop. This may make you feel dizzy.

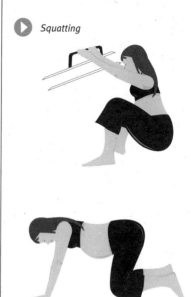

Squatting

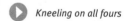

Kneeling on all fours

If you spend a long time in the tub, you must drink fluids, or suck on ice chips so that your body does not become too dry (dehydrated). During water therapy, your baby's heart rate will still need to be counted every now and then by your nurse or midwife. While you are in the tub, you and your labour coach can try some of the other techniques that make labour easier, such as massage, visualization, and special breathing.

Using your voice during labour

You may worry about crying out loudly during labour. Some women do, and others do not. Nurses, doctors, and midwives have heard women in labour making all kinds of sounds and noises. Many women vocalize during labour, others chant, moan, rock their bodies or heads from side to side, or cry. These are all normal ways to cope with labour. You should never feel embarrassed about using your voice during labour.

Transcutaneous electric nerve stimulation (TENS)

TENS is a safe way to manage pain. It does not use medicines. It sends small electrical impulses through electrodes placed on your belly or back to the nerves under your skin. TENS is thought to work in two different ways:

1. The electrical impulses block pain signals from going to the brain. For a woman in labour, the contractions may be causing pain, but your brain will not sense the pain.

2. TENS triggers your body to release more of the body's "feel good" hormone (endorphins).

If this method appeals to you, the physical therapy department of a hospital can arrange for TENS treatments. You should contact them before your labour, or speak with your health-care provider about using TENS during one of your prenatal visits.

Using medication for pain relief

Two main types of medicines are used to control pain during labour: painkillers and freezing.

- Painkillers are also known as analgesics. They dull the overall pain but do not make you lose all feeling in any part of your body.
- Freezing medicines are called anaesthetics. They cause a total loss of feeling in a certain part of your body.

We suggest you talk to your health-care team about the kind of pain relief you would like in your birth plan.

Painkillers (analgesics)

The most powerful painkillers are narcotics. You may be offered narcotics such as meperidine or morphine during labour. They are usually given by injection into the muscles of the hip, or sometimes through an intravenous (IV) line. They dull the pain and make you feel sleepy, so that you can rest between contractions. They may also affect your baby because they can cross through the placenta.

Narcotics are usually given only in the early and active stages of your labour, to make sure there is time for the effects to wear off before the baby is born. This helps to ensure your baby will be born alert and active. But if you need pain medicine and your baby is born "sleepy," the doctors and nurses can safely give her a medicine that will wake her up quickly so she is able to breathe on her own.

Freezing (anaesthetics)

An *epidural* is a common anaesthetic that blocks the pain of labour and birth. To get this medicine, a needle is inserted into a small space between the bones of your spine (vertebrae), and a doctor will inject the medicine into the groups of nerve endings found there. This numbs the nerves in that part of your body and blocks the pain.

When the doctor puts the medicine into your lower spine the first time, he will leave behind a small plastic tube (catheter) which will then be taped to the outside of your body. With this tube in place, you can receive more medication later.

Epidural medicine is often connected to a pump that provides you with a steady dose of the medication during labour. If you think you might want an epidural, it is best to discuss this with your health-care provider before you go into labour.

The medication in epidurals can be given to you in such a way that you can still have some control over your legs, can move into different labour positions, and can visit the bathroom. This is called a "light" or a "walking" epidural. For many women, it is the best option, as it still allows you to use and feel your body to help you with labour. You can also be in an upright position to help your labour along. You will probably be able to feel the urge to push and you may be able to do this better if you are not "frozen" from your epidural. Talk to your doctor (or anaesthetist) about this option.

Nitrous oxide

Nitrous oxide is an anaesthetic gas given through a face mask. You hold the mask and start breathing in the gas just before a contraction begins. It will give you some pain relief within two or three breaths. The effects will go away about five minutes after you stop breathing the gas. Nitrous oxide is very safe and does not make your baby sleepy.

The second stage of labour

The cervix is now open 10 centimetres and is fully dilated. The baby is ready to move down the birth canal. During the second stage of labour, contractions usually slow down. They happen two to five minutes apart and last about 45 to 90 seconds. This gives your body a much-needed rest between contractions.

Pushing

Most women feel an urge to push when their baby reaches a certain point in their pelvis. Pushing offers some relief from the "pressure" of labour. Pushing through a contraction has been described as a powerful release of stored energy that comes from deep within a woman's body and mind. You may feel powerful, strong, and in control when you begin to push.

When not to push

A couple of situations will delay pushing:

• if your cervix has not yet opened to 10 centimetres
• if your baby has not quite settled into the best position for pushing

Sometimes, the urge to push is so strong you simply cannot resist. With your nurse, midwife, or support person at your side to help you, you may be asked to put your knees very close to your chest and to use the "pant-pant-blow" method of special breathing until your cervix is fully open.

No urge to push

Some women do not feel the urge to push. They may need extra help and coaching to push their baby out. This may be the case for women who have had an epidural.

Some women go through a short time when they do not have any contractions, or their contractions are very light and they have no urge to push.

If your cervix is fully dilated, but you do not feel an urge to push—relax and rest for a bit. The urge will come in time. Sometimes, epidurals can affect a woman's ability to push, or can reduce the urge to push. Your nurse, doctor, or midwife will give you support and advice.

The natural rhythm of pushing

There is no right or wrong way to push. Although women are often encouraged to "take in a deep breath, hold it, and give one long steady hard push," studies show that this may not be the best method after all.

When women push naturally (without any instructions and based on their own rhythm), they tend to do three to five short pushes during each contraction. As the second stage of labour moves along, the number of pushes per contraction tends to increase. With natural pushing, women take in several big breaths of air with each pushing effort, and slowly blow all the air out of their lungs. Studies show that the natural way of pushing allows the most oxygen to reach your baby during the second stage of labour. Sometimes this natural way of pushing may take a few minutes longer.

Making room for the delivery

Often, a baby is born with little or no tearing of the perineum (the skin at the bottom of the vagina). The birth attendant may attempt to massage the skin around the perineum, helping it to stretch. About 70% of first-time mothers will need some kind of small and simple repair to their perineum after childbirth. While the tears are repaired, the doctor may freeze the area with a local anaesthetic to make you more comfortable.

Research has shown that such small tears heal better, with less pain, than a larger cut called an *episiotomy*. An episiotomy is a cut about 2.5 to 5 cm (1 to 2 inches) long. It is made at the bottom of your vagina toward the rectum or off to one side. Before making the cut, the doctor will freeze that part of your body with a local anaesthetic.

In some cases, an episiotomy is done to make more room for the baby's head and shoulders, or if it is important to speed up the delivery because of concern for the baby. An episiotomy should be done only if needed and depending on the situation at the time of the birth.

The third stage of labour

This stage of labour begins after the baby has been born and ends when the placenta comes out of your uterus (about 30 minutes after the birth). Other than having a few mild contractions to help push out your placenta, your work is done, and this is a time of relief.

As long as your uterus shrinks and stays firm (and there is no unusual bleeding), it is best to watch and wait for the delivery of the placenta.

If you need any repairs to your skin from tearing or an episiotomy, these repairs will be done after you have delivered the placenta. Finally, to help your uterus shrink and to stop the bleeding, your health-care provider is likely to give you an injection of oxytocin, a synthetic hormone. Studies show that routine use of this hormone after the baby is born will significantly reduce the amount of blood that a woman may lose after birth and can prevent too much bleeding (postpartum hemorrhage).

During this time, your nurse or midwife will feel the size and shape of your uterus to make sure that it continues to shrink and that the bleeding slows down. You and the nurses will be caring for your baby during this stage. You may tremble, feel chilly, or even feel like you may throw up (have nausea). The nausea should pass quickly and a warmed blanket will soothe your chills.

THE THIRD STAGE OF LABOUR

YOU CAN:

- *Relax. Hold and touch your baby.*

- *Provide skin-to-skin contact.*

- *Ask for a warmed blanket if you are shaky or chilled.*

- *Help push out the placenta when you are asked to do so (it is not painful to do so).*

YOUR LABOUR COACH CAN:

- *Bond with the baby.*

- *Help you get set up to breastfeed.*

- *Offer you something to drink, wipe your face and hands with a damp cloth.*

Handling your baby after birth

Once born, your baby will need to have the umbilical cord cut and clamped. The birth attendants will probably take a couple of minutes and will then dry your baby. At the same time, they will make sure that your baby has started to breathe properly and will begin to prepare for the Apgar score (see page 145).

Cord blood gases

Immediately after birth, a "cord blood gases" test is done. The health-care provider will take a sample of blood from a section of the umbilical cord after it has been cut; this is to check the oxygen and pH levels. The pH level measures the balance of chemicals in the baby's blood and is an important way to learn about the baby's well-being at birth.

The fourth stage of labour

The fourth stage of labour begins after the placenta is out and lasts about two hours. It is a time to rest, enjoy, and recover. During this time, you will be watched closely for any problems that may arise. Your nurse or midwife will check your blood pressure, heart rate, breathing, the position of the top of your uterus, and the amount of bleeding from your vagina. It is during this stage, as both you and your baby adjust to the changes of childbirth, that you will have your first chance to bond with your baby.

Bonding with your baby—Kangaroo Care

You and your baby should be together after the birth (don't forget to include your partner). You may want to keep your baby unwrapped and lying on your bare chest and belly, so that you have skin-to-skin contact. Nurses and midwives understand the bonding process and will support you to do this.

- They will dim the lights, so it will be easier for the baby to open his or her eyes.
- We suggest you hold your baby close, a few inches from your face, so the newborn can see you.

- Skin-to-skin contact is the best way to bond with your baby, and to keep the baby warm and comfortable right after birth. We call this Kangaroo Care.
- Talk quietly and softly using your normal tone of voice. You may notice the baby's face turning toward the sound of your voice and his or her eyes searching to make contact with yours.
- For the first hour or two after the birth, you will both be very alert. This is the best time for both bonding and the first breastfeeding. Breastfeeding your baby during this time will improve the way your baby latches onto your breast.

Over the next few days, use every chance you get to talk to your baby. Hold your baby close and continue to have as much skin-to-skin contact as you can. Handle your newborn slowly and carefully. Support the baby's head and neck and feed your baby whenever he is hungry.

Apgar score

A simple and quick method of testing newborn health is done one minute after the birth and again five minutes later. The Apgar score is essential to help health-care providers know whether your baby will need any special care. Five areas are rated during an Apgar score test:

1. the baby's heart rate
2. breathing
3. muscle tone
4. reflexes
5. skin colour

Each of these areas is measured and—depending on how the baby responds—rated from zero to two. Zero is the poorest response and two

NEWBORN SCREENING TESTS

All newborns are tested and screened to make sure they are healthy. Blood samples are taken in the first few days of life to test for disorders which can be present in a baby that seems to be healthy. All Canadian newborns are screened for health problems that affect how they digest food, how they produce hormones (which can affect normal growth and development), and for cystic fibrosis. The results will be sent to your health-care provider. You will learn of the results only if there are problems.

Screening for hearing is usually done while you are in the hospital and later, when your baby visits their health-care provider. These check-ups assess your baby's overall growth and development. If a hearing problem is found, a further test will be needed. Hearing problems can affect your baby's language and social skills.

is the best response. The total number of this test is the Apgar score. Most babies score between 7 and 10.

A baby who was born with a heart rate of 140 (scores 2), and a good strong cry (scores 2), with some movements (scores 1), coughing (scores 2), and pink all over (scores 2).

The total Apgar score, in this case, will be 9. Any Score over 7 at five minutes after birth predicts a healthy baby.

Apgar scores			
	score 0	*score 1*	*score 2*
Heart rate	*Absent*	*Slow (< 100 per minute)*	*> 100 per minute*
Breathing	*Absent*	*Weak*	*Good, strong cry*
Muscle tone	*Limp*	*Some movements*	*Active movements*
Reflexes	*No response*	*Grimace, whimpering*	*Cough or sneeze*
Skin colour	*Blue or pale*	*Body pink, arms and legs blue*	*Completely pink*

Special delivery: problems during labour and delivery

When labour may be induced

An overdue baby is only one reason for inducing labour. If your water breaks without labour starting on its own, you and your doctor or midwife will have to decide between inducing labour and waiting for it to start on its own. Either choice may be the correct one. It all depends on factors such as how long the membranes have been ruptured, whether the cervix is ripe (see page 147), the risk of infection, and your own feelings.

There are other reasons why it may be best to induce labour at 40 weeks of pregnancy or before. The reasons include:

• if the mother has high blood pressure that is getting worse
• if the mother has an illness such as diabetes

- if there are signs that the baby is not growing well
- if there are other medical concerns

Labour should be induced only for these valid medical reasons.

How labour is induced

There are several common ways to induce labour.

Ripen the cervix: Normally, the cervix begins to get softer, wider, and shorter before labour starts. This is called *ripening.* If your cervix is not getting ready for labour on its own, and you are having labour induced, your health-care provider may try to ripen your cervix. The most common way to do this is by placing a special gel or insert that contains a certain hormone (prostaglandin E2) onto your cervix or your vagina. Another way your health-care provider can ripen your cervix is by placing a rubber tube with a balloon on the end into the cervix and then blowing up the balloon. It is vital to soften or ripen the cervix before inducing labour.

Rupture the membranes: If the membranes of the amniotic sac are still in place, the next step may be to break them. This is done using a simple method: a specialized instrument is inserted into the cervical canal to puncture the membrane—the procedure feels like a routine examination of your vagina. For most women, labour will begin within 12 hours after the membranes are ruptured. This is most true if the cervix is also ripe. Some women have their membranes ruptured in order to speed up labour that has already started on its own, but without the membranes rupturing first.

Start the contractions: To bring about contractions of the uterus, your health-care provider can give you a drug called oxytocin, which is almost the same as the natural hormone you would produce.

Breech babies

Most babies are born head first. During the last month of pregnancy, they lie with their heads toward the birth canal. A baby is in a *breech position* when the baby's rear end is facing the birth canal.

If you are near your due date (the last four to six weeks) and your health-care provider suspects a breech baby, an ultrasound will be done to confirm the position, size, and health of your baby.

If the ultrasound confirms a breech position, you will need to discuss the choices for the best delivery. For some breech babies, the way their legs or head are sitting in the uterus will mean that a Caesarean section is safest. Other breech babies can be safely born through the vagina, as long as certain conditions are in place. You would need to discuss this with your health-care provider. A third option is to turn the baby to a head down position, using a technique called "external cephalic version" (ECV). After you have all the information you need and are aware of all the options, you can choose to have the ECV, a normal vaginal breech delivery, or a planned Caesarean section.

Assisted births: forceps or vacuum extraction

Sometimes, a baby needs to be helped out of the birth canal. A health-care provider may choose to assist the birth using **forceps** or a **vacuum extraction**. These methods are used when the second stage of labour has lasted a very long time, the woman is tired and is having a hard time pushing, but the baby is low enough to be born through the vagina with a little help. An assisted birth is also often used when a baby's heartbeat has slowed down—a sign that the baby may be in trouble.

Both forceps and vacuum extractor methods are common, safe, and very useful.

- **Forceps** are two slim, curved instruments that can slide around the baby's head inside the birth canal. Once they are in place, the doctor can adjust the position of the baby's head and help the woman's efforts to bring the baby down and out.
- The **vacuum method** is also called a "suction-assisted birth." It involves placing a plastic cup that is held in place by suction on top of the baby's head. A handle is attached to the cup. This allows the health-care provider to gently aid the baby's birth.

FORCEPS ASSISTANCE

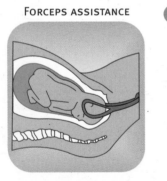

VACUUM EXTRACTION

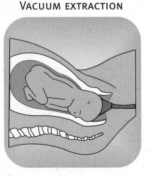

Caesarean births

A *Caesarean section* (also called a Caesarean birth or a C-section) is an operation that opens the pregnant woman's abdomen to remove the baby from the uterus. In Canada, about one-quarter of women have Caesarean births. Sometimes, for medical reasons, this surgery is planned in advance and done before labour begins. At other times, if problems arise for the mother or the baby during labour, it is done when labour is already in progress.

The most common reason for a Caesarean is "failure to progress in labour." Despite good and regular contractions, the cervix stops dilating for several hours or the baby fails to move down into the pelvis for birth. In these cases, and when all else has been tried without success, a Caesarean birth becomes necessary.

Concern about the baby's well-being is the second most common reason for a C-section. This happens most often when there are unusual changes in the baby's heart rate during labour. In most cases, this will need to be confirmed with a fetal scalp blood sample. If the health-care team strongly suspects that the baby may not be tolerating labour, and if the birth is not about to happen soon, a C-section will be considered.

The third most common reason for a Caesarean is the mother's history of having C-sections in the past. It used to be said that "once a Caesarean, always a Caesarean." We now know that this is no longer true. In fact, about 60 to 80% of women who have had a Caesarean birth before will now be able to give birth through the vagina.

If you had a C-section before, you should be aware that you have an excellent chance of having a vaginal delivery this time. Studies show that many women do not want to try labour again because they are afraid of having a long painful labour that will only end in another C-section. If this is how you feel, talk to your health-care provider. You need to know that you will have enough pain relief during labour.

Other less common reasons for C-sections include:

• the baby is in a breech position (see page 147)
• bleeding from a separated placenta
• bleeding from a placenta that covers the cervix

Sometimes a C-section is needed for the mother's health, as in the case of serious illness such as toxemia, or severe cases of diabetes. If a mother has an active herpes infection or HIV, the baby will be born by C-section to prevent the disease from spreading to the baby during the birth.

Childbirth is unpredictable. No one can fully control it, no matter how prepared they are. Whether you deliver your baby vaginally or by C-section, the goal of pregnancy is for you to become the mother of a healthy child. How you get to that goal is not as important as the goal itself. All women should be aware that a C-section may happen. When you create your birth plan, make sure you include what you would like to do if you need to have a Caesarean birth.

Many healthy babies are born by Caesarean to parents who are thankful that this safe way to give birth exists. Knowing that in an emergency you might need a Caesarean birth is a good reason to plan to have your baby in the safety of a hospital.

Postpartum hemorrhage

All mothers experience some bleeding after the birth, but 7 to 10% have postpartum hemorrhage, which is excessive bleeding. This is more common if the baby was large, if the labour was long and difficult, or if it was a multiple birth (twins or more). In the past, women died of this bleeding, but with modern medical care, postpartum hemorrhage is usually easy to treat.

How to prevent postpartum hemorrhage

Postpartum hemorrhage can be prevented. Recent studies show that giving women a hormone-like medicine (oxytocin) can prevent the risk of postpartum hemorrhage by up to 40%. Most hospitals now give this medicine to all women in labour, during either the second or third stage of labour. It is given by injection into a muscle or a vein.

Breastfeeding and massage of a soft uterus are two other good ways to prevent postpartum bleeding, because both stimulate the uterus to contract.

How long will you stay in hospital?

Benefits of going home early

You may be able to go home as early as a day or two after your baby's birth. Hospital stays have become much shorter in recent years. One reason is reduced spending on health-care, but the fact is: going home soon can be better for both you and your baby. You need to adjust to being a new mom. Your home is quieter and more relaxed than the hospital and you will likely sleep better in your own bed. You may have greater success with your efforts to breastfeed in the comfort of your own home, and your baby is less likely to get an infection. Also, it is easier for your partner and the rest of the family to spend time with the newest member of the family.

You should also know that maternity nurses and midwives are experts in teaching new mothers how to care for newborn babies. So, while you are in the hospital, we suggest you learn what you can from them. Do not be shy about asking all the questions you have about anything, even if you think the question may not be important. If it matters to you, it's important!

Follow-up home care

In Canada, we have the good fortune to have a public health system that provides follow-up home care after birth. The level of health care may vary from province to province. If you are going home early, it is very important that you have an early follow-up for the baby. This will be a home visit from a nurse or midwife.

Phone number for public health clinic:

_____

Date and time of first visit:

_____

Date and time of second visit:

_____

Nurse or midwife's name:

_____

*Things I need to ask the nurse or
midwife during my home visit:*

1. _____

2. _____

3. _____

4. _____

5. _____

6. _____

7. _____

8. _____

9. _____

10. _____

The Society of Obstetricians and Gynaecologists of Canada and the Canadian Paediatric Society have issued a combined statement about how to know when it is safe for mothers and babies to leave the hospital early (see the Postpartum Maternal and Newborn Discharge guideline at www.sogc.org). They clearly state that early home follow-up is essential to early discharge. By having a follow-up at home, you can be sure that feeding is well-established, that the baby is getting enough fluid and nutrition in his first days, and that jaundice is not a problem. Getting help early is important if your baby has any of these problems.

During a home visit, the nurse or midwife will examine you and your baby and answer your questions about caring for yourself and your newborn. The visit usually includes time to talk about your body, breastfeeding, diapering, baths, bonding with your baby, having sex again, and birth control. This private and close care will help give you the confidence you need to look after your new baby. It is a good idea to write your questions down before the nurse or midwife arrives, so that you will remember what you wanted to ask (see sidebar).

Longer hospital stays

Sometimes, it's best to stay in the hospital a little longer than usual. This may be the case if there were problems during the birth, if you had a long labour or a C-section, or if you or your baby need special attention or care. As well, a longer hospital stay may be important if your hospital does not offer a home care program or if you do not have enough support at home. Talk to your maternity nurse, midwife, or doctor if you have concerns about going home.

If things do not happen as you planned . . .

Despite modern medicine, babies are sometimes born with a serious illness or with problems the health-care team did not expect. It is very rare for babies to die. All parents hope for the best during pregnancy and most have bonded deeply with their unborn child before the birth. They begin to think of their baby as a person, as the newest member of their family.

It is a great shock when a baby is born with an illness, with genetic or physical differences, or without signs of life. Many mothers feel their bodies have betrayed them. They may feel they have disappointed everyone, including the baby and their partner. Some worry that they may have done something to make it happen. This is almost never true.

Parents can feel a deep sense of disappointment even if the baby is born alive, but with a serious illness or health problem. They feel grief because the child they imagined all through pregnancy does not exist. In some cases, it might take a while to adjust to a new baby with health problems. It may take time before all the challenges are discovered. There are many resources, both in the hospital and in the community, to help mothers and families adjust to life with a baby who has special medical or other needs.

Saying goodbye to a baby

The deepest and most profound sense of loss comes from the death of a baby. Many parents have trouble coping with their loss. Such a sudden tragedy causes intense sadness, shock, disbelief, and sometimes anger.

For parents and family, the grieving process is a necessary part of healing. Grieving helps parents cope. All parents can benefit from grief or bereavement support at such a tragic time in their lives.

Many hospitals have a service to help grieving parents. If not, a community health-care provider can help parents find resources to guide them through the grieving process. Sometimes, it helps if parents:

- Say goodbye by holding the baby. This will allow parents to create some positive memories. If the baby died because of birth defects, some parents may be afraid to do this, but in almost all cases, what the parents imagine is worse than it really is. Your health-care providers can help you decide if this is right for you.
- Hold a memorial service, a funeral, or a private ceremony.
- Talk about your feelings. Through many months of pregnancy, the baby has been a real part of your life. You can benefit from bereavement support to help you deal with your grief.

YOU AND YOUR PARTNER— SHARING THE LOSS

Your relationship with your partner may suffer from your shared loss. You may find you have trouble talking to, and even facing, each other. You may find it hard to do the normal things of life. It may be hard to start making love again. You may be angry with the other person and you may not know why. You may be searching for someone to blame. It is normal to feel this way.

Be patient with each other. Tell each other how you are feeling and be as open and honest as you can. Seek professional counselling. If your partner can't talk about the baby's death right now, remind yourself that you will be able to talk to each other about it in the future. Your baby is not forgotten. Everyone deals with grief in their own way and at their own pace. Make an extra effort to be tender and kind toward each other.

BABY'S BIRTHDAY

Date:

Time of birth:

Weight:

Length:

Hair colour:

Eye colour:

Health-care providers:

Notes:

My baby's journal

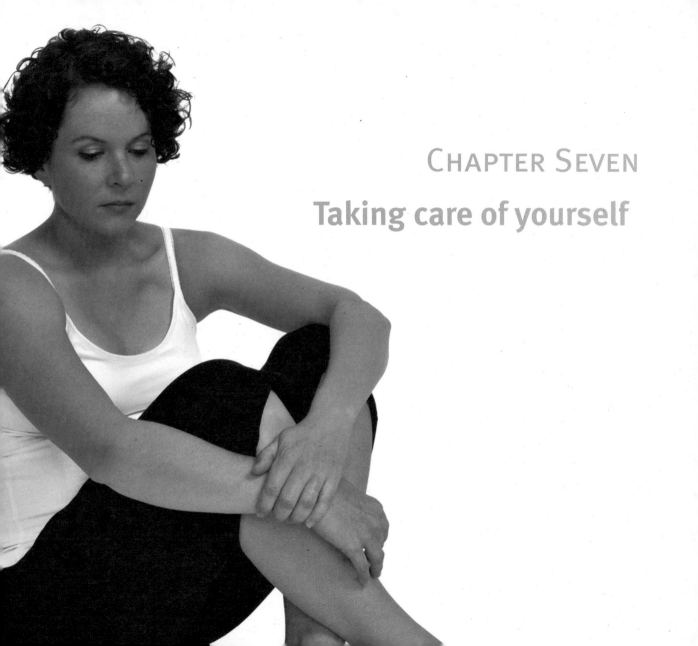

CHAPTER SEVEN

Taking care of yourself

RECIPE FOR REST

Many new mothers have a burst of energy right after their babies are born and then feel very tired. Your baby will be hungry every two to three hours for the first little while. You might begin to think all you do is feed your baby. Don't worry, your feelings are normal. Because regular feedings take a great deal of energy, you need to get lots of rest.

HERE IS AN EASY RECIPE TO REMEMBER:

R   **Relax** *whenever you can. Take a nap, read, watch television, and **sleep when the baby sleeps!***

E   **Eat** *well and drink plenty of fluids, especially if you are breastfeeding.*

S   **Share** *the responsibility of your new baby with your partner, family, and friends. Ask for help.*

T   **Take time** *to enjoy the baby. Let the housework wait (once in a while).*

Introduction

*Welcome to **your** chapter. Yes, you will have received lots of attention for the past nine months, but you have always had to share your body with your baby. Now, we're just going to talk about you. One of the most important things you can do for your new baby is to take care of yourself. Looking after a newborn is much easier if you are well-rested and healthy. Your body has just been through many months of change and stress.*

So, this is your chance to "get back on track"—a time when you can begin the physical and emotional healing you need after the stress and strain of your pregnancy. You should know right now that you will likely need about nine months to get your body back to where it was before your pregnancy. And you'll also be making some emotional adjustments—to the new member of your family and to the hormonal changes that come after birth.

It will take some work on your part. The good news is that you no longer have to go to prenatal appointments. Your first follow-up visit after birth will be about six weeks after the birth date. But, yes, you should still keep a journal until then. You may have heard about the "baby blues." We have a section on the subject. You may also have heard about "postpartum depression", which is different. We will cover that in this chapter. And after all the cautions and alerts about bleeding, and discharges, we have a couple of final concerns. On the happy side—sex? Your menstrual periods? Read on. We will also discuss some common discomforts and even birth control.

You will need time to get used to all the changes that come with having a baby. Now is a good time to ask for help from family and friends, and to accept their offers to cook meals, clean the house, do laundry, or babysit your other children. Take care of yourself.

Your changing body (postpartum)

The many changes your body went through during pregnancy happened slowly over nine months. In fact, it will take about the same amount of time for things to return to normal, so be patient with yourself.

After the delivery of your baby, you can feel your uterus if you press on your lower belly (halfway between your belly button and your pubic bone). Six weeks after birth, your uterus will almost be its normal size and you will not be able to feel it any more by pressing on your belly. Breastfeeding helps the uterus shrink back to its normal size more quickly.

The area between your rectum and your vagina is called your **perineum**. It will have stretched during the baby's birth. It may feel swollen, bruised, and tender. You may have stitches from a tear, or an episiotomy. These stitches will dissolve over time, but they can be itchy while they heal. Keep doing your Kegel exercises (see page 50) for more than six weeks after the birth. They will help the stretched muscles in your perineum regain their tone. Some women feel numbness in their perineum. This goes away over time.

The baby blues

After giving birth, it is normal to cry for no reason, to feel anxious, frightened, and sad. More than 70% of new mothers feel a little depressed after birth. For most women, this happens within a couple of days of the birth. You may have heard it called "the baby blues." It may be linked to the changing levels of pregnancy hormones, and may also come from feelings of loss, since the baby is no longer inside you. These feelings may last for hours or days. For most women, they go away within two weeks without any treatment.

You may feel a wide range of changing emotions. One minute you might feel happy, the next minute sad. You may feel very tired, and then get a burst of energy. You may have trouble sleeping, or making decisions. You

---

THE SIGNS OF POSTPARTUM DEPRESSION

- *My baby blues have not gone away after two weeks.*
- *I don't feel like my usual self.*
- *I have strong feelings of sadness or guilt.*
- *I often feel very anxious or worried.*
- *I have strong feelings of hopelessness or helplessness.*
- *I cannot sleep, even when I am tired.*
- *I sleep all the time, even when my baby is awake.*
- *I cannot eat, even when I am hungry.*
- *I cannot eat because I am never hungry, or because I feel sick.*
- *I worry about the baby too much; I'm obsessed with the baby.*
- *I do not worry about the baby at all; it's almost like I don't care.*
- *I am having anxiety or panic attacks.*
- *I feel angry toward the baby.*
- *I think about hurting my baby, or myself.*

If you have any of these signs, get help right away. If you know a new mother who has these signs of depression, get help for her. Counselling and treatment will help the feelings go away. Do not wait for things to get better. Call your health-care provider or your local crisis intervention line right away.

It's normal for the blood flow to slowly decrease with each passing day. If your flow has been decreasing, but suddenly becomes a lot heavier with bright red blood (which soaks through one or more maxi-pads within two hours and does not slow down or stop when you take time to rest), do not wait—go to a hospital immediately. If your flow has not fully stopped after six weeks, make an appointment to see your health-care provider.

It's not normal to:

- *develop large blood clots*

- *have an unusual discharge*

- *have a bad smell coming from your vagina*

If these things happen, it may mean you have a vaginal infection where you had an episiotomy or where you got the stitches. They can be serious and you will need to discuss what to do with a health-care provider.

may feel confident, then insecure. You may feel as though you will never get your old life or body back. You may not be interested in sex at all. All these feelings are completely normal. Now is when you reach out to your partner, family, and friends for support.

When "the blues" turn into depression

If the baby blues seem to be getting worse instead of better, or if they last more than two weeks, you may be moving into postpartum depression. This happens to a small number of new mothers. Some signs will alert you to seek help—and help is available.

You may feel sad. You may feel despair and think you are in a big black hole. You may have a sense of hopelessness. You may feel angry about "being on call 24/7." You may enjoy all the attention the baby receives, but feel jealous at the same time. You may feel in charge and then get angry that you have to be in charge. You may wonder if you are able to look after the baby and feel someone else would do a better job. You may feel frustrated or even angry when your baby cries. You may think he is crying just to annoy you. Thoughts or pictures may jump into your head about harming your baby or yourself. If you have any of these feelings – seek help immediately.

Postpartum depression is a clinical problem and you can talk to your public health nurse, your midwife, or your doctor about your feelings. It is not your fault. They will understand and be able to help you.

Normal vaginal discharge

Be prepared for a vaginal discharge after birth. It's called **lochia**, and is made up of blood and tissue from the lining of the uterus that your body will expel after birth. At first, the lochia is bright red and may contain a few small clots. Bright red blood may flow again for short periods during, or after, breastfeeding. This is because breastfeeding causes mild contractions in the uterus, helping to get rid of the lining. Also, blood may collect in the vagina while you are lying down and can gush out for a short time when you stand up. This is normal for the first few days.

Within a few days, your flow will begin to decrease and will become darker. As this happens, it is normal to notice some bloody spotting. Eventually, your flow will turn whitish or yellow and will slowly stop. This can last from 10 days to five weeks. If you are a second-time mother, your flow may not be the same as it was with your last baby.

If your flow is heavier than you think is normal, is heavier than a period, or if it smells bad, check with your health-care provider. It is best to use sanitary pads during this time, not tampons.

Having sex again

Having sex again is your choice. It's good to wait until you feel ready—at both the emotional and physical levels. Your body, mind, and spirit need time to adjust to the changes that childbirth and motherhood bring. If you are like most new mothers, you will likely be using all your energy to look after the baby. You may feel quite tired for the first few weeks.

Most couples do not have sex for four to six weeks after birth. It takes that long for your birth canal and uterus to resume their normal shape and size, and for you to feel comfortable. For some couples, the baby's demands make it hard to find the energy to have sex as often as before. Keep in mind that your partner has not been pregnant for nine months and may not be as aware of your physical (and emotional) condition as you are. So, you will both have to adjust to the changes a baby brings, which means TALKING—about BOTH your feelings (and frustrations too).

You may simply feel worn out by late-night feedings, all the excitement, and the added responsibility. You may also feel mildly depressed and not be interested in sex (part of the "baby blues"). But some new mothers feel insecure and do not like their body image and may not feel attractive for the first little while. All these feelings and worries are normal. If you have any concerns about starting to have sex again with your partner, make an appointment with your health-care provider for a check-up.

On the more physical side, please remember birth control (see pages 164 and 165 for birth control choices). You *can* get pregnant . . . again! If sexual intercourse is painful because of dryness, there are special jellies and creams to lubricate your vagina. You can also try changing positions to see if one is more comfortable than another. If you feel discomfort for a long time, talk to your health-care provider.

Common discomforts after giving birth

Tender breasts

When your milk comes in—about two to four days after the baby is born—your breasts may become very full, sore, and hard (see page 191 to learn more about engorgement). Breastfeeding your baby often helps drain the milk glands. Applying a warm compress to each breast may also be soothing. Using cold compresses between feedings and warm compresses for two to three minutes just before feeding may help.

If you are not breastfeeding, ice packs may help reduce the swelling. In most cases you do not need to empty or pump your breasts, since this will only make you produce more milk. If you are not sure if your baby is feeding well, talk to your health-care provider. Good support is important when your breasts are tender, and it helps to wear a good support bra, even at night. In some cases, your health-care provider may suggest pain medicine.

Vaginal pain

It's normal for the perineum (the area around your anus and vagina) to be swollen, bruised, and tender after you have given birth. For some women, this soreness lasts up to six weeks. If you have stitches, you may feel even more discomfort. Try this: wet and freeze a clean maxi-pad. Then put the frozen pad in your underwear. This should help reduce swelling. Sometimes a warm bath helps to get rid of the itching caused by healing stitches. Keep your vaginal area clean to avoid infection. Get plenty of rest with your feet up to take the pressure off. If you think you need pain medicine and you are breastfeeding, talk to your health-care provider. Some medicines can be passed on to your baby through your milk.

Cramping

Pains that feel like strong menstrual cramps are called ***after-pains***. They are caused by the uterus shrinking. They may feel worse during breastfeeding. First-time mothers may not feel after-pains. Try taking a warm bath, or put a heating pad across your belly. Pain medicine sometimes helps. The kind that you might take for menstrual cramps is likely the best choice. But always talk to your health-care provider before taking any medicine while you are breastfeeding. The deep breathing and relaxation techniques you learned during pregnancy may also help.

Bowel movements

You may not have a bowel movement for two to three days after the birth of your baby. The muscles in your abdomen that help you have a bowel movement have become stretched and do not work as well. Also, if you have not eaten very much, or if you had painkillers during or after your delivery, your bowels will be sluggish.

Do what you can to avoid hard stools, because they can cause hemorrhoids. Drink plenty of fluids and fruit juice, and eat foods high in fibre, such as bran muffins, bran cereal, fresh fruit, and vegetables. Stool softeners made with psyllium or natural fibre (such as coarse ground flaxseed) can be bought at the drugstore.

Hemorrhoids

Grape-like swellings around the rectum are called hemorrhoids. They are often painful and itchy. During a difficult bowel movement, especially with a hard stool, they may ooze a little blood.

As with vaginal or perineum problems, you can help reduce the swelling by freezing a damp maxi-pad and then putting it in your underwear.

Choose to lie down, rather than sit. This will take the pressure off your bottom until the hemorrhoids heal. There are special creams, sprays, and ointments that help shrink hemorrhoids. Talk to your pharmacist or health-care provider about what might work for you.

Problems with urinating

Right after the birth, or for the first day or so, you may find it hard to urinate. This is most true if you had a catheter or if you have stitches or a small tear in your vagina. To help the flow of urine get started, try turning on the taps in the bathroom sink so you can hear the water. To help take away the sting, urinate while taking a shower or a bath, or try squeezing warm water from a bottle over that part of your body when you urinate.

Later, you may find you have to urinate quite often or that you have trouble knowing when the urine is going to start flowing. You may lose urine with a cough, sneeze, or when you exercise. This problem is called **urinary incontinence**. It happens when the pelvic floor muscles get stretched—as they do during pregnancy and childbirth. You can help strengthen your muscles by doing Kegel exercises (see page 50). For most women, this problem slowly goes away.

Your body shape after pregnancy

The muscles in your abdomen stretched a lot during your pregnancy and they don't just spring back into place overnight once the baby is born. These muscles take time to slowly tighten back into their pre-pregnancy shape. During pregnancy, you gained weight slowly and it may take a few months to lose that weight. Do not try to lose weight quickly by eating a low-calorie diet. It's far better to eat a range of healthy foods and to resume exercise and increase it slowly over time.

Walking at a good pace is an excellent toning exercise. Push your baby in a stroller or carriage and your baby will enjoy it too. The latest weight-loss research shows that as little as 20 minutes a day of brisk walking or similar exercise will allow you to "burn" a lot of calories. If you restrict your diet in a severe way, the effect will be the opposite of what you want. Your body will adjust to famine by storing as much energy as possible in the form of fat.

In some communities, you may be able to find postnatal fitness classes that offer the fat-burning and toning exercises new mothers need. Joining these classes will give you a chance to meet other new mothers and talk about the things that are on your mind. If you are short of sleep and find that meeting all of your baby's needs is stressful, talking to other mothers about their lives and sharing tips on how to cope will help.

Not getting enough sleep and feeling stressed can raise the levels of a stress hormone called **cortisol**. This makes you store fat, especially around the midsection. Getting enough sleep is vital to losing weight.

Breastfeeding your baby will help you lose weight because your body burns extra calories to make breast milk.

Menstrual periods

If you are not breastfeeding, your menstrual period will start again four to nine weeks after the birth. Your period may be longer, shorter, heavier, or lighter than before pregnancy. It should return to what is normal for you after a few cycles.

If you are breastfeeding, menstruation may not start again for months, or until you stop breastfeeding altogether. However, your ovaries may begin to work before your period returns. This means you could become pregnant again without ever having your period. If you want to avoid pregnancy, you should begin using birth control as soon as you plan to be sexually active after the birth (usually four to eight weeks).

Birth control choices

If you do not want to get pregnant again right away, you and your partner should decide what type of birth control is best for you now. You *can* get pregnant while you are breastfeeding, even if your menstrual periods have not started again yet. So, now is a good time to decide which birth control method is right for you and your partner, and to have it ready before you begin having sex again. Talk to your health-care provider about your choices.

Breastfeeding: Breastfeeding will reduce (but not eliminate) your chances of pregnancy for the first six months after childbirth, especially if:

• you are breastfeeding often (at least every four hours, even at night)
• you do not give your baby formula or anything other than your breast milk
• you have not started your period again

As your baby grows older and starts eating other foods, breastfeeding becomes less frequent and your chances of getting pregnant rise.

The "pill," the "patch," and the "ring": All are hormonal contraceptives that work in a similar manner and must be prescribed by a health-care provider. The "pill" is taken orally (by mouth), the "patch" is applied to the skin, and the "ring" is inserted vaginally.

If you are not breastfeeding, you can begin using the "pill," the "patch," or the "ring" three to four weeks after your child is born. However, breastfeeding mothers should only use a particular type of birth control pill which does not decrease milk production. The progestin-only type pill (mini-pill) may be started immediately after delivery.

Injectable contraceptives (the "shot"): This is also a hormonal-type contraceptive. A health-care provider will give it to you in an injection once every three months. This form of birth control is safe, easy, and not too costly. Talk to your health-care provider to learn more.

Intrauterine device (IUD): Once your uterus has returned to its normal size—about six to eight weeks after birth—you can be fitted with an IUD in your health-care provider's office.

Latex condoms: Men wear this type of contraceptive. Condoms protect both partners from sexually transmitted infections. They are a good choice to have on hand.

Female condoms: Be sure to follow the instructions carefully.

Spermicides: They kill sperm and work best to prevent pregnancy when they are used with a latex condom. Follow the directions carefully.

Diaphragms or cervical caps: The opening to the uterus is covered by a diaphragm or cervical cap to prevent sperm from entering. If you used this method of contraception before you became pregnant, you will need to be fitted with a new one, but not until eight weeks after the birth. Diaphragms work best to prevent pregnancy when they are used along with spermicides.

To learn more, visit the SOGC's award-winning website at www.sexualityandu.ca

If you have completed your family—sterilization

Sterilization is a permanent birth control operation that can be done on both men and women. Although some sterilizations can be reversed, you and your partner should consider your decision carefully.

Vasectomy: Men can have this simple office procedure. It will be done by a urologist (a medical specialist) who cuts the tube (called the vas deferens) that carries sperm from the testicles. When this tube is cut, sperm cannot be delivered.

Tubal ligation: There are two ways to block the woman's fallopian tubes so that eggs cannot reach the uterus. One is an operation done in a hospital, usually under a general anaesthetic, by using clips or rings, or by burning the tubes. A newer method, done under local anaesthetic, uses small metal coils to block the tubes.

KEEPING TRACK OF MY PROGRESS
AFTER BIRTH (OR POSTPARTUM)

Date: _____

Blood pressure: _____

Weight: _____

THINGS TO DISCUSS WITH MY
HEALTH-CARE PROVIDER:

- *The baby blues—signs of postpartum depression*

- *Feelings about my baby*

- *Blood flow*

- *Feelings of pain*

- *Feelings about sex*

- *Birth control (contraception)*

- *Breastfeeding*

Other concerns:

_____

_____

_____

_____

My personal journal
Your follow-up visit

Your first follow-up visit is usually six weeks after the birth. Your baby will likely be checked two days after you leave the hospital and may be checked again weekly or a few times during his first month (see Chapter Eight).

_____

_____

_____

_____

_____

_____

_____

_____

_____

_____

_____

_____

_____

_____

_____

_____

_____

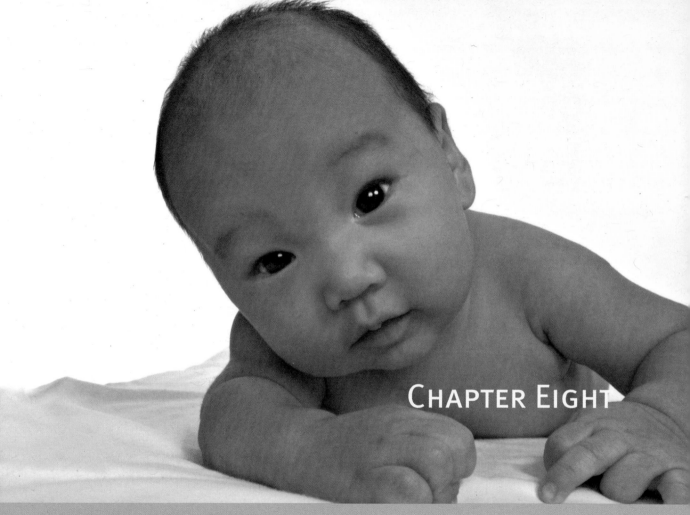

CHAPTER EIGHT

Taking care of your newborn

MAKE SURE YOU REGISTER
YOUR BABY'S BIRTH!

Every baby born in Canada must be registered. Ask your health-care provider how to do this, or contact Service Canada by phone at 1-800-622-6232, or through the Internet at www.servicecanada.gc.ca.

Aboriginal Canadians may want to look into the Indian Registration and Band Lists program. Information on this program can also be found on Service Canada's website.

Introduction

(Note: This chapter was reviewed by the Canadian Paediatric Society.)

As we begin this second-last chapter, congratulations are due—after all, you are now a parent! We hope we have helped answer your questions and prepared you well for the birth of your baby. We trust that you also received the support and help you needed from your support coach and health-care team. Canada is a great place to have a baby! The care you received from trained professionals is among the best in the world.

We will end this handbook with a few final details about your newborn that will help you start raising a healthy baby. There is lots of information available—just ask your health-care provider for suggestions—but we have found that parents (especially first-time parents) sometimes put so much focus on the birth that they may not be ready to care for the baby when it arrives.

So, as we've advised you how to care for your baby in the womb, we have new advice to take you through the first few weeks until you can get more information. For the most part, newborns eat, sleep, and are adored. Oh, and there are diapers, too.

*We will begin by telling you about how newborns look. Then, we'll cover some basic first care steps, vaccinations, and the choice of whether to circumcise or not. We'll also focus on diapers, feeding, and sleeping. Not that **your** child would cause trouble, but we also have a section for things such as colic. And, as with all other chapters in this handbook, we'll point out risks to your child.*

First impressions of your baby

Do not be surprised by some of the aspects of your baby's appearance at birth, and for the first few days. Newborn babies may have a waxy coating. When this is washed off, their skin may be a bit flaky from dryness. Many newborns have fine hair along their backs and shoulders. This usually goes away in a week or two. They may also have white spots, little bruises or marks, rashes, or blotchy skin; all these usually disappear with time.

During the journey down the birth canal, a baby's head may have been pushed into an odd shape. Over the next few weeks or months, the baby's head will come back to a more normal shape. You will also feel two soft spots—on the top and at the back of your baby's head (most parents only feel the top spot). These two spots are called **fontanelles** and they are places where the bones of the skull have not grown together yet. These soft spots are normal. Touching them will not harm your baby. In most cases, the bones of the skull grow together by the time a baby is 18 months old.

Some newborns have a full head of hair, while others have none. Some babies may lose their hair, only to have it grow back a different colour. The colour of your baby's eyes may also change over the next three to six months.

The hormones in your body at the time of the birth may affect your baby's body. For example, newborns of both sexes may develop swollen breasts when they are a few days old. Some babies' breasts leak a few drops of milk. Do not worry about this milk; it will go away by itself. Pregnancy hormones may also make the baby's sex organs larger than normal for a few days. A baby boy may have a reddish scrotum (the sac that holds his testicles), and a baby girl may have a bit of bleeding or white discharge from her vagina. All these symptoms are normal.

How to handle your baby safely

Your newborn baby may not be as fragile as you might think, but you do still need to handle your baby gently. This keeps him safe and feeling secure.

CARING FOR TWINS AND MULTIPLES

The birth of twins or multiples is an exciting event! You may have already done a lot to prepare yourself for the extra challenge of caring for more than one newborn. Changing diapers, breastfeeding, sleeping, doing laundry . . . all these tasks take on new meaning with twins or multiples. Ask for help. No one expects you to do it all yourself. Set up routines and patterns and then expect them to get broken! Take care of yourself. To learn more about being a parent to twins or multiples, see the Multiple Births Canada website at www.multiplebirthscanada.org.

MUSIC TO THEIR EARS

Start talking and singing to your baby as soon as she is born. She will love the sound of your voice and you will be creating a firm foundation for her language and literacy skills to build on as she grows.

Right from the moment they are born, newborn babies learn how to read signals all around them. They listen to voices, watch faces, and read body language. Babies need to hear and use sounds, sound patterns, and spoken language. This helps prepare them to talk and, eventually, to learn to read printed words.

When you hold your newborn baby, support the head. A baby's neck muscles are weak for the first few months of life. Even though the neck muscles are weak, the muscles in the rest of the body are quite strong! Strong enough to allow a squirming baby to move across a surface (where he could fall off), or to wave a fist, or push down his legs to knock a cup of tea or coffee out of your hand.

The best way to prevent any injury or harm is to watch, listen, and stay nearby. When you have to move away from your baby for any reason, put the baby in a safe place, such as the crib. Keep emergency phone numbers close to the phone, just in case. You may wish to take a class in baby CPR (Cardio-Pulmonary Resuscitation) so you will know what to do in case of an emergency.

Safety in your home

- Make sure all the equipment (such as cribs, strollers, and change tables) you have for your newborn meets national safety standards. Go around your house and do a baby safety check.
- Hang mobiles high enough so your baby's hands cannot reach them.
- Make sure that bookshelves or other pieces of heavy furniture are securely attached to the wall.
- Install a smoke alarm in your baby's room and make sure that all household smoke alarms are working.
- Never carry a baby and a hot drink at the same time.
- Do not heat any baby foods or bottles in the microwave. The microwave creates hotspots that can burn an infant's mouth. Warm a bottle in a pan of hot water instead and test the milk on your wrist before giving it to your baby.
- Never leave your baby alone with a pet.
- Supervise your baby around brothers and sisters and other young children.

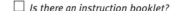

Safety around other people

Avoid crowds and crowded places with your newborn. Encourage everyone in your house to wash their hands before touching your baby. If they feel they must kiss the baby, ask them to kiss the top of the head instead of the face.

Safety when you are outdoors

Never leave your baby alone, whether in a car or a stroller or carriage. Do not use sunscreen or insect repellent on your newborn's sensitive skin. Instead, use an insect net and keep your baby in the shade. Use lightweight clothing that keeps skin and eyes shaded.

In the car

Always use a car safety seat, starting with your baby's first ride home from the hospital.

All infant and child car seats sold in Canada must meet Transport Canada's safety regulations. These rules help protect children in case the vehicle stops suddenly or is involved in a crash. Read the instructions that come with the car seat carefully. Put the seat into the car based on the instructions. The Universal Anchorage System (UAS) allows the baby's car seat to be installed with a seat belt in the rear seat of the vehicle. A forward facing seat will need to use a top tether strap. The best place for baby car seats is in the centre of the back seat, away from any airbags.

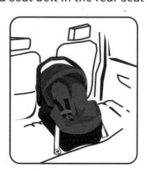

If you are having trouble setting up your infant car seat, contact your:

- provincial ministry of transportation,
- local public health unit,
- local police station. Some police forces offer free car seat inspections and clinics.

 Infant car seat

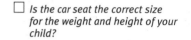

CAR SEAT SHOPPING CHECKLIST

☐ *Does the car seat have a national safety symbol?*

☐ *Is there an instruction booklet?*

☐ *Is the car seat the correct size for the weight and height of your child?*

☐ *If the car seat has an expiry date, will the time period cover your needs?*

☐ *Can the car seat be installed properly in your vehicle?*

☐ *Are the harness and tether straps easy to adjust?*

Source: Keep Kids Safe: Car Time 1-2-3-4, Transport Canada (TP 13511) www.tc.gc.ca/ roadsafety/tp/tp13511/tips.htm. Reproduced with the permission of the Minister of Public Works and Government Services Canada (2008).

 UAS symbol

You will find the UAS symbol on infant and child car seats, as well as on the vehicle seat next to the anchor bars and the place where you connect the car seat.

WHEN TO CALL YOUR HEALTH-CARE PROVIDER OR GO TO THE HOSPITAL

Do not wait! Call your health-care provider or find a way to go to the hospital safely right away, if your baby:

- *has a temperature of more than 38.0°C (100.4°F)*
- *has a seizure (shaking body, arms, and legs)*
- *has trouble breathing (works hard to suck air in, lips turn a blue/grey colour)*
- *has pale skin that feels cold and moist*
- *vomits more than twice in one day (large amounts of vomit, not the usual spit-up)*
- *has diarrhea (large watery stools) more than twice in one day*
- *passes blood or blood clots*
- *wets fewer than six diapers a day after the age of five days*
- *breastfeeds poorly or will not eat*
- *seems weak, can barely cry*
- *cries more than usual, cries in a different way, acts very fussy, and nothing you seem to do seems to comfort your baby*
- *does not act like he or she used to, seems "different" somehow, wakes up less alert, sleeps more than usual*

A healthy baby can become sick very quickly. If you are worried about your baby for any reason, call your health-care provider.

You should be careful about buying or borrowing a used car seat. Make sure it is not missing parts or instructions. You should never use a car seat that is more than 10 years old.

What to expect at your baby's first check-up

A baby's first wellness visit (or check-up) with a health-care provider should be within the first few days if you leave the hospital within 48 hours of the birth or if the baby is at risk of jaundice (see page 175). At this visit, your baby will have a complete physical exam. This includes measuring your baby's weight, height, and head size. Your health-care provider will also talk to you about the basic steps that babies go through as they grow. It's a good idea to bring a list of questions with you.

In many communities, a public health nurse contacts parents after the baby's birth to answer any questions and to set up a time for a home visit. During this visit, the nurse may provide you with information about taking care of both your baby and yourself. Many communities also offer Well Baby drop-in clinics where mothers and young babies can come without an appointment—a health-care provider can help direct you to such facilities.

Getting your baby immunized

Vaccines have been developed to protect babies and children from diseases that can cause serious illness, permanent suffering, or death. Vaccines that are offered to your baby through the public health system are very safe and effective. It's important to make sure your child receives these vaccines at the right times so he can be protected.

Below is a schedule of immunizations that will be offered to your child. The schedule may vary slightly from province to province. Talk to your health-care provider if you are planning to move from one province to another. Together, you can make sure that your child will not miss any vaccines.

Routine childhood immunization schedule (2006)										
Age at vaccination	Diphtheria Tetanus Pertussis Poliomyelitis	Hib[1]	Mumps Measles Rubella	Tetanus Diphtheria Pertussis	Hepatitis B[3]	Chickenpox (Varicella)[4]	Pneumococcal	Meningococcal conjugate[5]	Flu	HPV[6]
Birth					Infancy or			Infancy 1, 2, or 3 shots depending on age or adolescence	6–23 months 1–2 doses	
2 months	X	X					X			
4 months	X	X					X			
6 months	X	X					X			
12 months			X			X	X			
18 months	X	X	X[2]							
4–6 years	X		or X[2]							
9–13 years					X					X
14–16 years				X						

Notes:

1. *Haemophilus influenzae* type b (Hib) requires a series of immunizations. The exact number and timing of each may vary with the type of vaccine used.

2. A 2-dose program for MMR exists in all territories and provinces. The second dose of MMR is given either at 18 months or at 4 to 6 years of

VACCINE SAFETY IN CANADA

- *The vaccines used in Canada are very effective and safe.*

- *Serious negative reactions are rare. The dangers of getting the disease itself are many times greater than the risks of serious reactions to the vaccine.*

- *Health authorities around the world are very serious about making sure vaccines are safe.*

- *Expert committees in Canada investigate reports of serious negative effects.*

- *There is **NO** evidence that vaccines cause chronic disease, autism, or sudden infant death syndrome. The links that some people say happen—for example, between hepatitis B vaccine and multiple sclerosis—have been proven to be false after scientific study.*

Source: Canadian Immunization Guide, 6th Edition (2002), p. 45, http://dsp-psd.pwgsc.gc.ca/Collection/
H49-8-2002E.pdf, Public Health Agency of Canada. Reproduced with the permission of the Minister of Public Works and Government Services Canada (2008).

age. If the child is past the age when the second MMR is recommended, the second dose can be given 1 to 2 months after the first.

3. Hepatitis B requires a series of immunizations. In some parts of the country, this series may be given at a younger age.

4. Given in one dose to children between 1 and 12 years old and in two doses, one month apart, for older children. It is not recommended for children under 1 year old.

5. The recommended schedule and number of doses depends on the age of the child. There are five different types of meningococcus that cause infection in humans. Type C vaccine is now given routinely to babies. A new vaccine that covers types A, W-135, Y and C is also available. This vaccine is not currently recommended for routine use in Canada. It is used for people at higher risk of getting meningococcal infection. It is not covered by provincial or territorial public health plans.

6. For girls only. The second dose is given two months after the first, and the third dose after six months.

If you have Internet access, you can go to the Public Health Agency of Canada's website to learn more about immunization, to get the most up-to-date schedule, and to find the schedule that applies to the province where you live: www.phac-aspc.gc.ca.

Source: Canadian Paediatric Society, www.caringforkids.cps.ca.

Common questions about vaccines

Are vaccines safe?

Yes. Vaccines are very safe. Serious side effects are rare.

Why do we need vaccines if the diseases they prevent no longer exist?

Most of the diseases we are vaccinated against do still exist both in Canada and in countries where fewer people are immunized. Outbreaks of the disease do occur.

Why can't I take a chance that my child will not get sick?

Children who are not vaccinated have a much greater chance of getting the disease than those who have received the vaccine.

Do vaccines weaken the immune system?

No. Vaccines make the immune system stronger to protect against certain diseases.

Can natural infection be an alternative to vaccines?

Vaccines create immunity to certain diseases without making a person suffer from the disease itself. Many of the diseases children are vaccinated against can kill or disable them, so we want to prevent as many people as possible from getting the natural disease.

Jaundice (yellowish skin and eyes)

Most jaundice is not harmful to your baby. The physical signs of jaundice include the skin and the whites of the eyes turning a yellowish colour. **Jaundice** is caused by the build-up of a substance in the baby's blood called bilirubin. Jaundice usually appears during the first 3 to 5 days of life. It goes away as the baby's body becomes able to deal with the bilirubin. A health-care provider can check for jaundice by doing a blood test that measures the bilirubin in your baby's bloodstream. This blood test may have been done before you left the hospital with your baby.

If you leave the hospital 24 to 36 hours after giving birth, a health-care provider should check your baby on day two or three for jaundice. In many centres in Canada, a nurse does this on an early home visit. If you do not have this service in your community, you can arrange to have your baby checked by a health-care professional in a clinic.

EMERGENCY AND COMMUNITY CONTACT NUMBERS:

MEDICINES FOR NEWBORNS

Talk to your health-care provider before you give your baby any:

- *herbal remedies*

- *vitamins*

- *over-the-counter drugs*

While many are sold without a prescription and are deemed safe, some substances can be harmful, especially to newborns. ALWAYS check with your health-care provider first.

It is uncommon for babies to have such high levels of bilirubin that they are in danger, but if you think your baby has jaundice:

- Feed the baby based on the feeding cues or every 2 to 3 hours during the day and night.
- Call your health-care provider.

Most babies do NOT need hospital treatment for jaundice. If they do need treatment in hospital, they will be put under special lights (phototherapy) to reduce jaundice.

If your baby is jaundiced and dehydrated (see "Signs of dehydration in newborns" sidebar on page 178), irritable, has low energy, is arching her back, or has shaking movements that seem like a seizure, go directly to a hospital emergency room.

Circumcision

Circumcision is an operation to remove the skin that covers the head of the penis. An infant must be stable and healthy to be circumcised. After a careful review of the medical evidence, the Canadian Paediatric Society does NOT support circumcision as a routine procedure for newborns. However, many parents decide to circumcise their sons for personal, religious, and cultural reasons. Since circumcision is not essential for health, you should make a decision based on your own values, while knowing the benefits and risks.

If you choose not to circumcise, it's important—and easy—to keep the uncircumcised penis clean. You just need to wash the area gently while you are giving him a bath. The foreskin does not fully pull back (retract) for several years and should never be forced back. Later, when the foreskin fully retracts, your son should be taught to wash gently under it.

Circumcision is an operation that creates some discomfort for the baby. It also carries some risks. After circumcision, you should contact your health-care provider if:

• your baby does not urinate within six to eight hours
• bleeding lasts for a long time
• you notice redness around the tip of the penis that gets worse after three days

Cord care

The stump of the umbilical cord usually shrivels up and falls off in a week or two. The spot under the stump will become the baby's belly button. Just use plain water to clean your baby's cord stump. Avoid any other liquids.

To keep the cord dry, fold the top of the diaper away from the stump. If the skin around the cord becomes red or swollen, smells bad, or has pus coming out, the cord may be infected. Call your health-care provider if you think your baby's cord is infected.

Eye care

After the baby was born, the nurse placed special drops (or an ointment) in the baby's eyes to prevent infection from germs that may have entered the eye during the birth. Unless signs of infection appear—such as redness or a discharge from the eye—all you need to do to keep the area clean is wipe each closed eye with a moist cloth. If you think the baby's eyes are infected, call your health-care provider or the public health nurse.

SIGNS OF DEHYDRATION
IN NEWBORNS

Dehydration (when the body's fluid levels drop) can be very serious. Call your health-care provider right away or find a way to go to the hospital safely right away. Do not wait if you notice any of these signs in your baby:

- drowsy, sleepy, hard to wake up

- less urine (wets less often, or diapers are not as wet). Your baby should have 6 to 10 wet diapers each day

- dark yellow urine

- still passing meconium, or dark stools, on day three or later

- dry mouth, lips, or tongue

- weight loss of more than 10% in the first few days

- any fever

Newborn care

Your baby's elimination system

Elimination is essential for your baby. You can tell if this body system is working well by the number of times your baby soils or wets the diaper (see table on page 179). Newborns can get dehydrated very quickly. Dehydration is a drop in the baby's fluid levels. This can cause serious problems. That's why it's very important to feed your baby often—at least 8 to 12 times a day in the first few weeks—and to make sure your baby has normal amounts of urine and feces, the waste that comes from having a bowel movement (also called stool).

Your baby's first bowel movement will look a bit like tar. It will be greenish-black. It's called **meconium**.

- Babies pass meconium for the first day or two after they are born.
- After that, your baby's stool will become looser and greenish-yellow for three to four days. This is called transitional stool.

If your baby's urine is almost clear and hard to see in the diaper (but you can still feel the diaper is wet or heavier than a dry diaper), this is a good sign that your baby is getting enough milk. Very yellow urine may mean your baby is dehydrated and needs more milk (fluids). Make sure you check the diaper every time you change your baby to make sure it is wet. If there is plenty of fluid going in, then plenty of fluid (urine) should be coming out.

Newborns who lose more than 10% of their total body fluids can become very ill. Know the signs of dehydration in newborns (see the sidebar on this page). Call your health-care provider if you have any concerns.

Your health-care provider will want to know:

- the number of soiled and wet diapers your baby has had
- the amount and colour of the stool you see in the soiled diapers

Baby's Age	Wet Diapers *How many, how wet*	Soiled diapers *Number and colour of stools*
1 day	At least 1 **WET**	At least 1 to 2 per day **Black or dark green**
2 days	At least 2 **WET**	
3 days	At least 3 **WET**	At least 3 per day **Brown, green or yellow**
4 days	At least 4 **WET**	
5 days 6 days 7 days 2 weeks 3 weeks 4 weeks 5 weeks	At least 6, pale yellow *or clear urine* **HEAVY WET**	At least 3 large per day, soft and seedy **Yellow**
6 weeks to 6 months		At least 1 or more every 1 to 7 days **Yellow**

Skin care and bathing

Your baby must be kept clean, but you do not need to give a full bath every day. A warm cloth will help keep the baby clean between baths. Wash the face and hands often. Clean the area inside the diaper after each diaper change.

It's all right to give your baby a bath even if the cord has not fallen off. You may use mild baby soaps to clean the skin. Use a moisturizing cream to soothe dry skin. Pay special attention to the scalp and the folds in the baby's skin. For safety reasons, it is best to use a baby bathtub. Do not use your adult bathtub or a bath seat or tub ring in your regular tub. These are not safe for infants.

SAFETY TIPS FOR CHANGING DIAPERS

1. Gather all the items you need **before** you lay the baby down to be changed.

   You will need:

   • *small washcloths or disposable baby wipes*

   • *a clean diaper and maybe clean clothes*

   • *ointment to prevent diaper rash*

2. Never turn your back on your baby, not even for a second!

3. Put your hand on the baby's tummy if you must reach for something. If you cannot reach what you need, take the baby with you.

4. Ignore the doorbell or phone if they happen to ring. Or take the baby with you to answer them.

5. Avoid using baby powder that can be inhaled by the baby.

6. Wash your hands after each time you change your baby, to prevent germs from spreading.

7. Keep the surface where you change the baby's diapers clean.

DIAPERS AND YOUR BABY

Since newborns wet up to 18 times a day and have bowel movements as often as 10 times a day, you will need to have plenty of clean diapers on hand. To keep your baby's skin clean and dry, change your baby each time the diaper is dirty. Most parents find a routine for changing diapers that works for them. For example:

- *Some parents change the baby after each feeding and before they lay the baby down for a nap.*

- *Others find that changing their baby's diaper is a good way to wake up a sleepy baby that still needs to breastfeed from the other breast.*

Having a good routine for changing diapers will help prevent diaper rash.

Bathe your baby in a warm room. Gather all the items you will need first, and take off any jewellery you are wearing that might scratch the baby. Fill the basin with about two inches of warm water and test the water using the inside of your wrist to make sure it is not too hot. Hold your baby securely during the bath.

Use clean water to wash the eyes, ears, mouth, and face. Do not use cotton swabs to clean inside a baby's nose or ears. You can use a clean washcloth wrapped around your little finger to clean the outer ear and nose. Mucus or earwax will come out by itself in time. Do not use baby oil. It can make your hands and the baby's skin slippery and unsafe.

Start at the top, and work your way down. Wash the face first, then the body, then the bottom. Wipe a girl's genitals from front to back. You do not need to separate the vaginal lips. Keep a baby boy's penis clean by gently washing the area. Do not try to pull back the foreskin—it's usually not safe to do this until a boy is at least 3 to 5 years old.

After you take the baby out of the water, pat your baby completely dry with a towel. Never leave a baby alone in a bathtub, even for one second.

Trimming fingernails and toenails

Keeping your baby's nails short will help prevent scratches to your baby's face. Little mittens or small socks on your baby's hands will also prevent scratches, but it's just as easy to cut her nails. Carefully cut the nails straight across, using fine scissors or baby clippers. You may find it easier to file the nails at first, instead of cutting them. The best time to cut a baby's nails is when she's sleeping.

Dressing

Babies need the same layers of clothing as their parents are wearing. In the winter, they may need an undershirt, a shirt, and a sweater, along with warm clothing on their legs, socks or booties, and a snowsuit. In the summer, they may be most comfortable in only a T-shirt and diaper.

In air-conditioned rooms or cars, your baby may need more clothes than you do, because he is less active. Babies tend to feel cold sooner than you would.

Choose clothing with safety and comfort in mind. Make sure sleepers are snug and there are no drawstrings that could get caught on hooks or knobs. Make sure snowsuits are not so big that they prevent you from making the car seat buckles as tight as they should be, or make it possible for your baby to slip out of the car seat.

Common skin rashes

Your newborn baby may have some skin rashes or spots that do not seem to be normal to you. Most are very common and do not need to be treated.

Baby acne is a red, pimply rash on the face. It usually goes away over time.

Milia are tiny whiteheads on your baby's face. They will also go away over time.

Erythema toxicum is a common splotchy red rash that tends to come and go on different parts of a newborn's body. It is most common on the second day of life, but can appear at birth or within the first two weeks. Each splotch might have firm yellow or white bumps surrounded by a flare of red. They may stay for only a few hours, or for several days. They will slowly disappear.

Cradle cap looks like crusty patches on the baby's scalp. There might be some redness around the scales and on other parts of the baby's body—such as in the folds of the neck, armpits, behind the ears, on the face, and in the diaper area. This usually goes away on its own.

Diaper rash is a red rash in the diaper area. It is caused when urine or stool in the diaper makes the baby's skin tender and red. You can help prevent diaper rash by changing your baby's diaper often. (See "How to prevent diaper rash" in sidebar on this page.)

HOW TO PREVENT DIAPER RASH

- *Change your baby's diaper often.*

- *Keep your baby's diaper off for short periods. This gives the skin a chance to dry and helps prevent and treat mild cases of diaper rash.*

- *When you are changing your baby's diaper, use mild soap and warm water to wash the area well. Wipe from front to back. Rinse and let the skin fully dry before you put a new diaper on.*

- *Apply unscented petroleum jelly or a cream made with zinc oxide to the skin of the diaper area. This will protect the skin and add moisture to it.*

- *Wipes can dry out a baby's tender skin. If you use them, make sure they are alcohol-free and unscented.*

- *Avoid using baby powder or talc. It can be inhaled by the baby.*

Source: Canadian Paediatric Society, www.caringforkids.cps.ca.

Swaddling is a way of wrapping your baby to make them feel safe and secure. It can help settle and calm your baby. Some babies like to be swaddled with their arms out so they can move them around. Stop swaddling when your baby is about one month old or when she begins to kick off her covers. This is the time when babies want and need to move around more.

Here's how to swaddle your baby:

1. *Check that your baby is not hungry or wet before you start.*

2. *Place a cotton crib sheet on a flat surface and fold down the top right corner about 15 cm.*

3. *Place your baby on his back with his head on the fold.*

4. *Pull the corner near your baby's left hand across the body, and tuck the leading edge under the right arm and around under the back.*

5. *Pull the bottom corner up under your baby's chin.*

6. *Bring the right-hand corner over and tuck it under the back on the left side.*

Candida diaper rash appears around the genitals and buttocks and is made up of small very red spots on top of larger red patches. It is a type of yeast infection that can also appear in the baby's mouth. When it's in the mouth, it's called **thrush.** If you think your baby has a candida infection, see your health-care provider. Candida rashes need to be treated with a prescription cream.

Heat rash usually happens during hot and humid weather, or in winter if your baby wears too many layers of clothing. It causes little red bumps on the skin—mostly in the folds of a baby's skin or on parts of the body where clothing fits snugly. You can help prevent or treat heat rash by taking off extra clothing and by keeping your baby cool by dressing him in loose-fitting, light cotton clothing (especially in warm, humid weather).

Contact dermatitis is a rash that occurs when your baby's skin comes into contact with something that irritates the skin, or something that he is allergic to (such as snaps on clothing or dyes in clothing). In most cases, it only appears on the part of the skin that came in contact with the item your baby is allergic to. Tell your health-care provider if this happens. Finding the cause of the rash may involve taking a careful history of things the baby is exposed to.

Eczema is a skin rash that shows up as dry, thick, scaly skin, or tiny red bumps that can blister, ooze, or become infected if they are scratched. It appears most often on a baby's forehead, cheeks, or scalp, but it can also spread to other parts of the body. It may happen in babies who have allergies or a family history of allergy or eczema. There is no cure for eczema, but it can be controlled and often will go away after several months or years. Talk to your health-care provider if you think your baby has eczema.

Ways to prevent a flat head

Babies who always sleep on their back with their head to the same side can develop flat spots. This is not dangerous and will not affect a baby's brain or development. In most cases, it goes away on its own. But you can also prevent your baby from getting a flat spot by changing the placement of your baby's head each day. You can:

• Place your baby with the head at the top of the crib one day so that she must turn in one direction to look out into the room.
• The next day, place her head at the foot of the crib so that she must turn her head in the other direction to look out into the room. Change your baby's direction in the crib each day.
• Have "tummy time" when the baby is awake, several times a day. You must supervise your baby at all times! Lay your baby on her tummy while you are present and talking or singing to the baby.

Sleeping in a safe environment

Your baby needs lots of sleep to stay healthy, happy, and growing. So where your baby sleeps is important. If you create a safe place for your baby to sleep, you will reduce the risk of injuries and the risk of **Sudden Infant Death Syndrome (SIDS)**. SIDS is when a baby under 12 months old dies unexpectedly while sleeping. No one knows what causes SIDS, but studies show that there are some simple things that you can do to help reduce the chances of SIDS (see sidebar on this page).

For the first six months, the safest way for your baby to sleep is on her back in a crib, in your room. This also makes it easy to do night-time breastfeeding, and may help protect against SIDS.
Source: Canadian Paediatric Society, www.caringforkids.cps.ca.

Roommates or bedmates?

Your baby in a crib in your room is an excellent set-up because you are close and can breastfeed easily without actually sharing a bed. Adult beds are not designed for infants. They can be unsafe because:

WAYS TO REDUCE THE RISK OF SUDDEN INFANT DEATH SYNDROME (SIDS)

• *Put your newborn to sleep on his back, on a firm, flat surface. When your baby is old enough to turn over onto his tummy, then you do not need to make him sleep on his back.*

• *Make sure there are no fluffy pillows, comforters, blankets, duvets, stuffed toys, or bumper pads in the crib. These things could cover the baby's face and hinder breathing.*

• *Use clothing that will keep the baby warm but not too hot, even when they are sick. Sleepers should fit snugly.*

• *Do not smoke or use alcohol or drugs around your baby.*

• *Never put your baby on a waterbed.*

• *Breastfeed your baby. It's healthy and natural and may protect against SIDS.*

Adapted from the Canadian Paediatric Society's position statement "Recommendations for Safe Sleeping Environments for Infants and Children" (2004) and parent handout "Safe sleep for babies." Available at www.caringforkids.cps.ca.

BREASTFEEDING IS THE MOST
HEALTHY AND NATURAL WAY TO
FEED YOUR BABY

REMEMBER:

The colostrum you produce in the first day or two after giving birth is the perfect food for your new baby. Although your breasts produce only a small amount of colostrum, it is enough. You do not need to give your baby anything else.

• A baby can get trapped between the mattress and the wall or the bed frame.
• A baby can fall off the bed.
• An adult or older child can roll over and suffocate a baby.
• Soft bedding can cover the baby's head and cause overheating or suffocation.

Feeding your baby

The time you spend feeding your baby is a special time for both of you. Babies thrive on being held close. They also love to suck and love the feeling of being full of warm milk. Many new mothers feel a close bond forming with their babies when they feed them.

The Society of Obstetricians and Gynaecologists of Canada, the Canadian Paediatric Society, the United Nations Children's Fund (UNICEF), and the World Health Organization (WHO) recommend breast milk as the best and only food for babies for the first six months. After six months of only breastfeeding, parents can begin to give the child other foods, while still breastfeeding (until your child is two years old or even older). Breast milk contains antibodies, growth factors, enzymes, and other things that affect your baby's short- and long-term health. No type of formula has these benefits.

Babies who receive formula will have the basic nutrition to grow. However, parents should be aware of some of the increased health risks that come from using formula. There is the risk of infection from bottles, nipples, and utensils that must be washed properly when you prepare the formula. Parents should know how to prevent infection and how to prepare formula safely (see page 193 for details on cleaning bottles, pumps, and other equipment).

Breastfeeding

Breast milk, including the colostrum of the first few days, is the natural food for infants. It has all the right ingredients in just the right amounts to help them grow. It is the perfect temperature, does not cost anything, and is always available. As well, breastfeeding helps you to lose weight, and helps your uterus to shrink back to its normal size. Breastfeeding helps you feel close to your baby.

At first, your breasts produce **colostrum**. It is a yellowish sticky milk-like substance rich in vitamins, protein, and antibodies to protect your baby from infections. Newborns have fat and water stored in their bodies. They use this up in the first day of life. This explains why newborns lose weight at first. Colostrum alone is enough food for your baby for the first few days. There is no need to give your baby water or formula. The amount of milk you produce will increase within two to three days.

Eating balanced meals and drinking fluids is important while you are breastfeeding. Do not diet. You will slowly lose weight. Remember that it took nine months to gain the extra weight during pregnancy. It will likely take nine months to lose it and return to your pre-pregnancy weight.

When to start

The best time to start breastfeeding is within the first 30 to 60 minutes after giving birth, when your newborn is very alert and ready to suck. Your nurse will ask if you want to breastfeed your baby, and will help you to get started. Skin-to-skin contact helps both you and the baby with two important things: bonding and breastfeeding.

Not all babies learn how to breastfeed right away. It is still a good idea to use this time to get breastfeeding started. Make sure you let the hospital staff know that you want your baby to stay in your room with you (rooming in) so you can breastfeed your baby whenever he seems hungry. Feeding your baby often helps to increase your milk supply.

VITAMIN D

Babies need enough vitamin D to promote healthy growth. Not having enough vitamin D is called vitamin D deficiency. Babies at risk for this are those who:

- *are only breastfed*
- *are not exposed to enough sunlight*
- *have darker skin*
- *live in northern communities (north of 55 degrees latitude, about the level of Edmonton)*

If a baby's mother does not have enough vitamin D, the baby will also be at risk of the same problem. All babies at risk should get a daily supplement of vitamin D.

While breast milk is the best food for a growing baby, it only has small amounts of vitamin D. It may not have enough to meet a baby's needs.

- *Babies who are breastfed should get a daily supplement of 400 IU of vitamin D per day from birth until they get enough from the food they eat.*
- *Babies in northern communities or who have darker skin should get 800 IU per day between October and April when there is less sunlight.*

Talk to your health-care provider or community health nurse about your child's vitamin D needs and how to meet them.

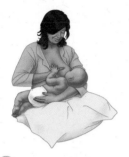

Cradle hold

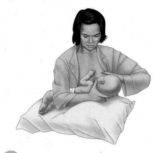

Cross cradle hold

Adapted and reproduced with permission of Public Health, Region of Peel.

Breastfeeding positions

You can breastfeed your baby in many comfortable positions. Here are a few suggestions:

Lying down

Lie in bed on your side, with your head on a couple of pillows. Lay the baby down beside your lower breast.

Cradle hold

Find a comfortable sitting position. Prop a pillow under the arm that holds your baby. Put the baby's head at your breast with the baby's feet lying across your abdomen.

Cross cradle hold

Find a comfortable sitting position. Prop a pillow under the arm that holds your baby. Support your baby at the base of his head and neck using the arm opposite to the breast that will be used. Support the baby's back and buttocks with your forearm. Your baby's ear, shoulder, and hip should be in a straight line with his stomach touching your stomach.

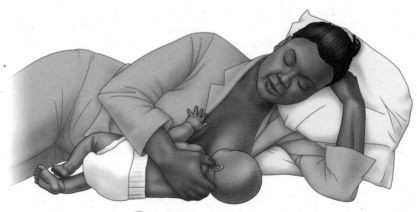

Lying down

Adapted and reproduced with permission of Public Health, Region of Peel.

Football hold

Find a comfortable sitting position. Tuck the baby's legs under your arm so the feet point toward your back. Use a pillow to support the baby's head at the level of your breast. (This position puts less pressure on your abdomen if you had a Caesarean birth.)

How to get started

Step 1. Get comfortable

Use pillows to support your arm. Hold the baby close and point the face toward your breast. Bring the baby toward you. Do not go toward the baby. If you do, you may have back pain and an uncomfortable latch.

Step 2. Latching on

Getting a good "latch" is the most important part of breastfeeding without discomfort. Here are some tips to help you:

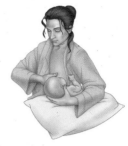

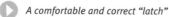 *Football hold*

Adapted and reproduced with permission of Public Health, Region of Peel.

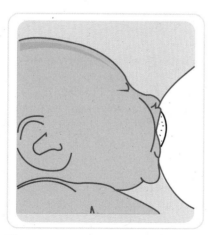

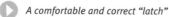 *A comfortable and correct "latch"*

- Roll your baby's body toward you and wait until her mouth opens.
- Point your nipple toward the baby's nose. When bringing the baby toward your breast, support her neck and shoulders. Do not push on her head. Once the baby is latched, the chin—not the nose—will touch your breast.
- Put your baby onto the breast with the lower jaw well down on the areola (the dark area around the nipple) and lots of your nipple in the mouth.
- This way, your baby will not be sucking from the nipple, but applying pressure with the jaws and tongue further back. This will allow milk to flow from the milk ducts around the nipple into her mouth. You will be able to see your baby swallowing the milk.

Step 3. Breaking the suction

To take the baby off your breast, slide your smallest finger inside the corner of the mouth and push down gently to break the suction seal. Do this every time you want to take the baby off your breast to prevent your nipples from getting sore. Then go back to Step 2 and try to get the baby to latch on again.

Breastfeeding tips

- Make sure your baby is latching on in the correct way and that you feel comfortable during breastfeeding before you go home from the hospital. Ask for help if needed.
- Be sure to drink water often during the day.
- Get into a comfortable position before you begin breastfeeding.
- Being skin-to-skin with your baby in the early days will help the breastfeeding process.
- Keep your baby close to you so you can see and hear his feeding cues as soon as possible.
- Burp your baby after each feeding.
- Start with one breast, letting the baby breastfeed for as long as he likes.
- The baby will fall asleep, stop sucking, or let go of your breast when finished.

- If your baby falls asleep too quickly on your breast, try using breast compression to help him to drink more.
- Make sure that your baby is not too hot (wearing too many clothes) while breastfeeding.
- Take a break. Burp your baby. Change a soiled diaper and wash your hands. (This often helps the baby to wake up and continue feeding.)
- Start again with the other breast. If he won't take any more, try to remember to start with this breast next time.
- Try starting with a different breast at each feeding.
- You can feed your baby from both breasts each time, or you can feed him from one breast one time and the other breast the next time. Either way is perfectly fine. The more milk that flows from the breast at each feeding, the more milk you will make.
- Feed your baby often at first to help the amount of milk increase and to prevent your breasts from being engorged (see page 191).
- Some babies have growth spurts around 3, 6, and 12 weeks. They will ask to be fed more often for 24 to 48 hours. This is nature's way of helping you to produce more milk.
- Taking care of a newborn is tiring. If possible, ask for help with the baby, housework, and other children.

 Expressing breast milk

Expressing breast milk

Learning how to hand express your breast milk is important. You can do this when you want to rub a few drops of milk on your nipple, to soften your areola, or to store milk to let someone else feed when you cannot be with your baby.

- Wash your hands, get comfortable, and have a clean or sterile container ready to collect the milk.
- Massage your breasts with both hands.
- Place your thumb and first finger on the edge of the areola while supporting your breast with the rest of your hand.
- Push gently back toward your chest wall.

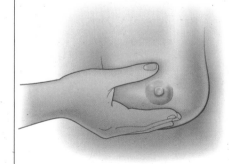

Adapted and reproduced with permission of Public Health, Region of Peel.

Expressing breast milk

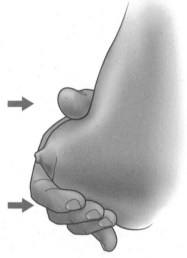

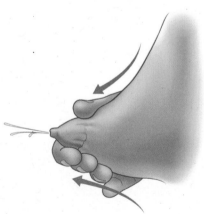

• Roll your fingers and thumb toward the nipple while you also apply slight pressure.
• Release the pressure and repeat this step in a rhythmic motion.
• Continue until the flow of milk has slowed down or stopped.
• Rotate your hand to empty all areas of the breast then repeat all steps with the second breast.

Don't worry if you only get a few drops of milk at first. This skill becomes easier and more efficient with practice. You can also express your milk using a manual or electric breast pump.

Seal the container that contains your breast milk. Put a label on it with the date and time. You can store breast milk safely in these ways:

• at room temperature for about 6 hours,
• in the refrigerator for 3 days,
• in the freezer of your refrigerator for about 3 months, and
• in a chest freezer for about 6 months.

Common breastfeeding problems

Tender, sore breasts

Wearing a full-support breastfeeding bra that fits you well, even at night, may help. Change breastfeeding positions to remove milk from all parts of your breasts. Make sure both breasts get a balanced amount of breastfeeding time. The best way to care for your breasts is to make sure that your baby latches on the correct way and that you are comfortable, every time.

Sore nipples

During the first couple of weeks of breastfeeding, it is common for your nipples to feel tender when your baby first latches on to the breast. You will likely notice this tender feeling as the baby latches on. It will reduce by the time you count to 10. Once the baby is latched in the correct way and you feel comfortable, there should be no pain. If you have nipple pain throughout the feeding or after the feeding, this is a sign that something might be wrong.

Check with the hospital nurses or your public health nurse to be sure your technique is good. Make sure the baby latches on the correct way and that you feel comfortable. If not, break the seal and get the baby to latch on again. Breastfeed often, offering the breast as soon as the baby first seems hungry. Crying is a late hunger cue—by then, the baby may be too hungry to get a good latch.

To help heal the nipples, spread a few drops of breast milk over them and let them dry in the air after each feed. Breast milk contains fats that help heal and protect the skin of the breasts. Modified lanolin cream may also be helpful. Use unscented soap for daily washing. If you use breast pads to absorb leaking milk, make sure you change them often so that they do not leave your nipples damp.

Engorgement

Breastfeeding involves supply and demand. Breasts become **engorged** (hard, lumpy, and painful) when the supply of milk is greater than the demands made by the baby. After a while, your breasts learn how much milk is needed to keep your baby satisfied and well fed and they will not produce more than that. That's why it's important to feed your baby often and not to miss any feedings. Engorged breasts can sometimes be so swollen that the nipple becomes flat. This makes it very hard for the baby to latch on to. In this case, you will need to express some milk to take the pressure off the breast and allow the flattened nipple to stand up. If your breasts become engorged and you do not provide relief, you may end up with a lower milk supply. Get help to make sure that your baby is latched on in the correct way and that you feel comfortable.

To reduce engorgement, use a cold compress on each breast between feedings. If you want to improve milk flow, use warm compresses and massage just before feeding begins.

Blocked milk ducts

You may have a blocked milk duct if you notice one area of a breast that seems more tender, warm, and swollen. If so, it is best to try to open the milk duct before breastfeeding by putting warm compresses on your breasts. Then massage your breasts in an effort to move the milk toward your nipples as you breastfeed your baby. Start under your arms. Make sure the baby latches on in the correct way and that you feel comfortable. Breastfeed your baby as often as you can to help keep the milk flowing. After the feeding, put cold compresses on your breasts to reduce swelling.

Mastitis

Mastitis is an infection of one or more milk glands in the breast. It may happen when milk does not empty fully from the breast. Women can prevent most cases of mastitis by:

- learning how to get a good latch so your baby is taking the maximum amount of milk from each breast;
- breastfeeding on demand, as often and for as long as your baby wants;
- breastfeeding exclusively, without giving any other fluids or food in the first six months;
- expressing enough milk to feel comfortable if your breasts feel full or engorged after a feeding.

You should check your breasts often to see if any lumps are forming, or if there is any pain, hotness, or redness. These may be early signs of mastitis. If you do develop mastitis, you may feel like you have the flu (with fever and chills) and you may notice a reddened hot spot on one or both breasts. Call your health-care provider right away and have the position of the baby and the latch assessed right away to make sure the baby is truly taking milk from the breast.

Mastitis is a serious infection that can be treated with antibiotics. Get plenty of rest. It is important to continue to empty milk from a breast with mastitis. Take pain relief and continue to breastfeed as usual. A baby can feed from a breast with mastitis; it is not harmful. If you find it is too painful to breastfeed your baby from the breast with the infection, you should try to remove milk from your breast using gentle hand expression or a breast pump.

What if I cannot breastfeed?

For some mothers, breastfeeding is not an option. Sometimes your health-care provider may suggest formula feedings for medical reasons. This kind of feeding will provide your baby with the needed calories and nutrients.

It is important to choose the right formula for your baby and to prepare it correctly. To learn more about choosing and preparing formula, talk to your health-care provider, contact your local public health office, or go to www.bchealthguide.org.

Cleaning bottles, pumps, and other equipment

You may use pumps, bottles, or other infant feeding equipment if you are expressing breast milk. All must be cleaned carefully before you use them. Wash the equipment well in hot, soapy water and rinse off the soap. Leave it to air dry.

If your baby is preterm or sick, sterilize the equipment. To do this:

• Submerge the equipment in a deep pot of water.
• Bring the water to a boil, and let it boil for 10 minutes.

Spit up

Most babies "spit up." It happens during or after a feeding when the contents of the baby's stomach goes back into the tube that connects the mouth to the stomach. Spitting up tends to peak at 4 months. Most infants stop spitting up by about 12 months of age.

▶

Never, never shake your baby!

Shaking can damage your baby's brain. It may even kill him. No child should ever be shaken.

WALK AWAY

CALL FOR HELP

However, if you notice any of these signs in your baby, speak to your health-care provider. It may be a sign of Gastroesophageal Reflux Disease (GERD).

- Vomit combined with blood or green or yellow fluid, or poor weight gain.
- Severe crying and irritability.
- Refusing food and gaining very little weight.
- Breathing problems (such as not taking full breaths, turning blue, chronic cough, wheezing, or having pneumonia more than once).

Why babies cry

Colic and crying

Healthy babies cry. It is the way they express their needs and communicate with the people around them. Most of the time, parents respond with what their baby needs by offering food, helping the baby sleep, changing a diaper, or just cuddling. If you look at it that way, crying is quite useful for babies who depend on other people to meet all of their needs.

But there are times when even the most caring parent cannot soothe a baby's cries. Be aware that it's not your fault.

When a baby cries long and hard (without a break) even though he has been fed, changed, and cuddled, the baby is said to be "colicky." For a long time, people thought that colic was a health problem that some babies had and others did not.

But new information suggests that what used to be called colic is really a normal part of being a baby. All babies go through a time early in life when they cry more than at any other time.

Each baby is different. During this time of heavy crying—which happens most often between 3 and 8 weeks—some babies may cry much more than others. Their crying may seem stronger, and it may be harder (sometimes impossible!) to soothe.

The good news? First, it is normal. And there is no lasting effect on your baby. Second, it will not last forever. This time of intense (and unexplained) crying can end as quickly as it started, or it may slowly decrease over time. In most cases, it ends by the time your baby is 3 to 4 months old.

In the meantime, there are some tips to help you get through a stressful time. (Refer to section below "What can parents do to help soothe a crying baby?")

Why do some babies cry more than others?

Some experts believe that babies who cry more than others are just more sensitive by nature and have a hard time controlling their crying. They may have more trouble soothing themselves and getting settled into their natural body rhythms when they are very young.

In general, studies show that there is nothing wrong with the bowels of babies who cry long and hard. Nor is there strong evidence that the crying is caused by gas, wind, or food allergies. In fact, crying causes infants to swallow air, which they burp up or pass as wind. Because they strain and tighten their stomach muscles, this also forces air out of the rectum.

What can parents do to help soothe a crying baby?

Each baby is unique, and what helps soothe one baby may not work for others. The challenge for parents is to find what works for their baby. Be aware that there may be times when nothing works even though you try everything. This does not mean you are a bad parent.

Here are some suggestions that might calm your baby or help to prevent crying at times when your child is fussy:

• Check to see if the crying is a sign that your baby needs something—a diaper change, a feeding, relief from being too hot or too cold, or attention for a fever.
• Hold your baby. This will not spoil him. However, some babies do not like being passed from person to person.

- Wrap or swaddle your baby in a soft blanket.
- Turn off the lights and keep the room quiet. Too much noise or action can often trigger crying or make it worse.
- Soft music, or a gentle shushing noise can soothe some babies.
- Many babies are soothed by motion. Try walking with your baby in a sling or in a stroller. Rock or sway the baby in a gentle, rhythmic motion. Or try going for a ride in the car.
- Sucking sometimes helps babies to calm down and relax. You can provide this by breastfeeding or by offering a pacifier.
- Give your baby a warm bath.

Although there are reports of some over-the-counter and natural remedies being helpful for colic, talk to your doctor before using them.

Only do gentle and soothing things to comfort your baby. Never shake your baby. If you are feeling upset by the crying or feel frustrated that your best efforts are not helping, put the baby in a safe place (like her crib) and take a moment to calm yourself.

Call your doctor if:

- Your baby is not behaving as usual and is not eating or sleeping.
- Your baby has a fever, is vomiting, or has diarrhea.
- Your baby could be hurt from a fall or injury.
- Your baby cries excessively after 3 months of age.
- You are afraid you might hurt your baby.

Where can you go for help?

The early days of taking care of a new baby can be difficult. You may not be sleeping much and you might be trying to meet your baby's needs 24 hours a day.

A baby's constant crying can be stressful. The most important thing to know is that it is not your fault. And it will get better. In the meantime, be sure to take care of yourself.

Arrange for child care relief so you can get some rest. Find a friend, family member, or someone else you trust who can look after your baby for short periods while you get a break. If people offer to help, accept their help.

- It sounds simple, but eating and sleeping well can make a big difference in how well you can cope. Try to get at least 3 hours of sleep in a row, twice a day.
- Sometimes you may have negative thoughts. That's okay, as long as you do not act on those thoughts. If you feel depressed or angry, talk to someone you trust and get help.
- Many community resources offer support to parents, especially new mothers. If you are not sure where to go, talk to your pediatrician, family doctor, or public health nurse.

Source: Canadian Paediatric Society, www.caringforkids.cps.ca.

What about pacifiers (soothers)?

Throughout history, parents have used pacifiers to help comfort and calm their babies. Scientific studies have linked the use of pacifiers with dental problems, ear infections, and early weaning from breastfeeding. On the other hand, pacifiers offer comfort to babies during painful procedures and have been linked to lower rates of SIDS. If you choose to use a pacifier, take this advice:

- Avoid using one until breastfeeding is fully established.
- Never use a pacifier instead of feeding, comforting, or cuddling the baby.
- Make sure the pacifier is clean and not damaged.
- Never dip the pacifier in sugar or honey.
- Never tie a pacifier around your baby's neck.

(Adapted from the Canadian Paediatric Society, "Pacifiers (soothers): A User's Guide for Parents." For more information on soothers and other tips about caring for your baby, go to the Canadian Paediatric Society's website for parents at www.caringforkids.cps.ca)

Parenting classes

Classes to promote good parenting skills are offered in most communities. These classes are good for every new parent because they help boost your knowledge and confidence. The best thing they offer new parents is a chance to share their experience with other parents who have many of the same problems and joys. The classes are very useful and helpful for first-time parents, and for very young new parents.

In these classes, you will learn basic parenting skills, such as feeding, how to change a diaper, and bathing. You'll also talk about other topics, such as child safety, sibling rivalry, and coping with frustration. If you and your partner came to Canada not long ago from another country, parenting classes may help you learn more about raising a child in Canada.

First aid and infant CPR (Cardio-Pulmonary Resuscitation) courses are also available. To learn more about these courses and how to register, contact the Canadian Red Cross or your public health centre.

Here we are, at the end of our role—getting you through your pregnancy and off to a positive start. So, please accept our best wishes for a long healthy life for you and the newest member of your family. Happy baby!

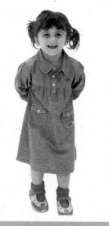

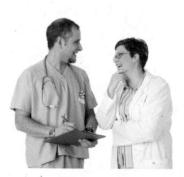

CHAPTER NINE

Finding help

Key resources and services

Most people have questions about pregnancy and the growth of their baby. This section provides key resources and services about your health, before and during pregnancy, and in the first few weeks after your baby is born. The list includes helpful websites, documents, programs, and phone numbers that will help you find answers to your questions or learn more about having a healthy pregnancy and baby.

The Society of Obstetricians and Gynaecologists of Canada: Pregnancy Resources

The SOGC is a national medical society in the field of sexual reproductive health. The society promotes excellence in the practice of obstetrics and gynaecology and works to advance the health of women through leadership, advocacy, collaboration, outreach, and education.

Birth Plan
Sample birth plan.
www.sogc.org/health/pregnancy-birth-plan_e.asp

Clinical Practice Guidelines
www.sogc.org/guidelines/index_e.asp

Cord Blood Banking
www.sogc.org/health/pregnancy-cord-blood_e.asp

Due Date Calculator
www.sogc.org/health/pregnancy-calculator_e.asp

Group B Streptococcus Infection in Pregnancy
www.sogc.org/health/pregnancy-groupb_e.asp

Herbal Remedies
www.sogc.org/health/pregnancy-herbal_e.asp

Multiple Births
www.sogc.org/health/pregnancy-multiple_e.asp

Nausea and Vomiting During Pregnancy
www.sogc.org/health/pregnancy-nausea_e.asp

Preterm Labour
www.sogc.org/health/pregnancy-preterm_e.asp

sexualityandu.ca
This website provides Canada's one-step source for information and education on sexual and reproductive health, contraception, and sexually transmitted infections.
www.sexualityandu.ca

Ultrasound in Pregnancy
www.sogc.org/health/pregnancy-ultrasound_e.asp

Vaginal Birth After Caesarean Section
www.sogc.org/health/pregnancy-vbac_e.asp

Aboriginal Resources

Aboriginal Clinical Practice Guidelines
www.sogc.org/guidelines/index_e.asp

Aboriginal Nurses Association of Canada
The only Aboriginal professional nursing organization in Canada.
1-866-724-3049
www.anac.on.ca

Aboriginal Tobacco Strategy
The purpose of this website is to promote "tobacco wise" Aboriginal communities.
www.tobaccowise.com

Canada Prenatal Nutrition Program
Community-based services provide food, nutrition information, support, education, referrals, and counselling on health issues.
www.phac-aspc.gc.ca/dca-dea/programs-mes/cpnp_main-eng.php

Canadian Aboriginal AIDS Network
This non-profit coalition of people and organizations provides leadership, support, and advocacy for Aboriginal people living with and affected by HIV/AIDS, no matter where they live.
1-888-285-2226
www.caan.ca/english/home.htm

First Nations, Inuit, and Aboriginal Health
Health Canada information on First Nations people and Inuit to improve their health.
http://www.hc-sc.gc.ca/fniah-spnia/index-eng.php

Institute on Aboriginal People's Health
*Supports research to address the
special health needs of Canada's
Aboriginal people.*
www.cihr-irsc.gc.ca/e/8668.html

Irnisuksiiniq—Inuit Midwifery Network
*This network aims to keep midwives
and maternity care workers up to
date on midwifery events and
resources.*
1-877-602-4445 ext. 252
*www.naho.ca/inuit/midwifery/index
-e.php*

**National Aboriginal Health
Organization**
*Promotes the well-being of First
Nations, Inuit, and Métis people.*
1-877-602-4445
www.naho.ca/english

**National Association of
Friendship Centres**
*A central unifying body for the
Friendship Centre movement.
Promoting and advocating for the
concerns of Aboriginal
Peoples, and representing
the needs of local
Friendship Centres.*
www.nafc.ca

Pauktuutit: Inuit Women of Canada
*Fosters greater awareness of
the needs of Inuit women,
advocates for equity and
social improvements,
and encourages participation
in the community, regional,
and national life of Canada.*
1-800-667-0749
www.pauktuutit.ca/home_e.asp

Abuse (Violence) Resources

Domestic Violence 24-hour hotline
1-800-363-9010

Shelternet—Shelters for Abused Women
*Website connects abused women to
shelters.*
www.shelternet.ca

Alcohol and Drug Use Resources

*All provinces and territories have
programs for people with alcohol and
other drug problems. Ask your health-
care provider.*

Alcohol and Pregnancy
*The Public Health Agency of Canada's
website provides information about
alcohol and pregnancy.*
*www.healthycanadians.gc.ca/hp-gs/
know-savoir/alc_e.html*

Alcohol-Free Pregnancy
*The Best Start Resource Centre's
website provides information about
alcohol and pregnancy.*
1-800-397-9567 ext. 260
www.alcoholfreepregnancy.ca

Canadian Centre on Substance Abuse
*Provides access to a range of
information for substance abuse issues.*
1-613-235-4048
www.ccsa.ca

Motherisk
*Information and guidance for pregnant
or breastfeeding women about risks
associated with drug, chemical,
infection, disease, and radiation
exposures. Information on alcohol and
substance use in pregnancy.*
1-877-327-4636
www.motherisk.org

Bereavement (Grief) Resources

**Canadian Foundation for the
Study of Infant Deaths**
*Information about Sudden Infant
Death Syndrome (SIDS) and
bereavement.*
1-800-363-7437
www.sidscanada.org

Parentbooks
*A full selection of books on fertility,
pregnancy and birth, pregnancy
and infant loss, infant and child
development and parenting.*
1-800-209-9182
www.parentbooks.ca

**Perinatal Bereavement
Service Ontario**
*Support services for perinatally
bereaved families.*
1-888-301-7276
www.pbso.ca

Child Health and Development

About Kids Health
*The Hospital for Sick Children—
AboutKidsHealth website
provides families with reliable,
current information about all
aspects of child health and
family life in a format that
is easy to understand.*
www.aboutkidshealth.ca

Best Start Resource Centre
*Online resources about
prenatal care and
child health.
1-416-408-2249
Toll-free within Ontario:
1-800-397-9567
www.beststart.org*

**Breastfeeding Committee for
Canada**
*Protect, promote and support
breastfeeding in Canada as the
normal method of infant feeding.
www.breastfeedingcanada.ca*

**Canadian Association of Family
Resource Programs**
*Parenting resources, including a
directory of family resource programs
across Canada.
1-866-637-7226
www.frp.ca and
www.parentsmatter.ca*

**Canadian Coalition for Immunization
Awareness & Promotion**
*Information about immunizations for
all ages.
1-613-725-3769 ext. 122
www.immunize.ca*

Canadian Immunization Guide
*Lists the immunizations that are
recommended in Canada.
www.phac-aspc.gc.ca/publicat/cig-gci/
p03-01-eng.php*

Caring for Kids
*Child and youth health information
from the Canadian Paediatric Society.
1-613-526-9397
www.caringforkids.cps.ca*

**Centres of Excellence for Children's
Well-being**
*This website provides recommendations
on the services needed to ensure the
best early childhood development.
1-514-343-6111 ext. 2525
www.excellence-earlychildhood.ca*

Growing Healthy Canadians
*Information on how to promote the
well-being of children and youth.
www.growinghealthykids.com*

Infant Care
*The Public Health Agency of Canada's
webpage provides information about
infant care.
www.phac-aspc.gc.ca/dca-dea/
prenatal/index_e.html*

Invest in Kids
*Resources and programs for parents.
1-877-583-5437
www.investinkids.ca*

La Leche League Canada
*Information and support for
breastfeeding.
1-800-665-4324
www.lllc.ca*

Mother Goose Program
*This group program uses rhymes,
songs, and stories to nurture the
parent-child relationship.
1-416-588-5234
www.nald.ca/mothergooseprogram*

Nobody's Perfect Parenting Program
*Offers an education and support
program for parents of children from
birth to age five.
www.phac-aspc.gc.ca/dca-dea/family_
famille/nobody_e.html*

Oral Health for Children
*Health Canada—children's oral health
care information.
www.hc-sc.gc.ca/hl-vs/oral-bucco/care
-soin/child-enfant_e.html*

Peel Region Health Department
*Information and short video clips
about breastfeeding.
www.peelregion.ca/health/family-
health/breastfeeding/first-weeks/
index.htm*

Child Safety

Car Seat Information
*Ontario Government information about
choosing and installing car seats.
www.mto.gov.on.ca/english/safety/
carseat/choose.htm*

Car Seat Safety
*Transport Canada information sheets
about car safety for children.
1-800-333-0371
www.tc.gc.ca/roadsafety/safedrivers/
childsafety/car/index.htm*

Safe Kids Canada
*The national injury prevention
program of SickKids works with
partners and parents across Canada
to reduce unintentional injuries and
deaths.
1-888-SAFE-TIPS
www.safekidscanada.org*

**The Centre of Excellence for
Child Welfare**
*Promotes child welfare research,
policy development, and knowledge
dissemination.
www.cecw-cepb.ca*

Children with Special Needs

Your public health nurse can help if you think your baby has a developmental problem or a disability. Most communities have an infant development program for children. Staff in this program can help you with activities for your baby that will encourage development. They can also help you find support services.

Autism
Autism Society Canada.
1-866-476-8440
www.autismsocietycanada.ca/index_e.html

Canadian Down Syndrome Society
1-800-883-5608
www.cdss.ca

Canadian National Institute for the Blind
A primary source of support, information and, most important, hope, for all Canadians affected by vision loss.
1-800-563-2642
www.cnib.ca

Centre of Excellence for Children and Adolescents with Special Needs
Ensures that young people with special needs living in rural and northern communities receive the best services Canada has to offer.
www.coespecialneeds.ca

Health-Care Providers

Society of Obstetricians and Gynaecologists of Canada
The SOGC is a national medical society in the field of sexual reproductive health. The society promotes excellence in the practice of obstetrics and gynaecology and works to advance the health of women through leadership, advocacy, collaboration, outreach, and education.
1-800-561-2416
www.sogc.org

Association of Women's Health, Obstetric and Neonatal Nurses Canada
Promotes the health of women and newborns.
1-800-561-2416 ext. 266
www.awhonncanada.org

Canadian Association of Midwives
The national organization that represents midwives and the profession of midwifery in Canada.
1-514-807-3668
www.canadianmidwives.org

Canadian Association of Nurses for Women and Newborns
Canadian, bilingual voice for nurses caring for women, newborns and families.
www.canwn–aicfnn.ca

Canadian Fertility and Andrology Society
Promotes study and research about infertility.
1-514-524-9009
www.cfas.ca

Canadian Nurses Association
The national professional voice of Registered Nurses.
1-800-361-8404
www.cna-nurses.ca

College of Family Physicians of Canada
National voluntary organization of family physicians.
1-800-387-6197
www.cfpc.ca

Doula C.A.R.E.
Information about Doulas, and a list of Doulas.
www.doulacare.ca

The Royal College of Physicians and Surgeons of Canada
To locate certified medical specialists who are Fellows of the RCPSC.
www.royalcollege.ca

Health Information—General

Health Canada
www.hc-sc.gc.ca

Public Health Agency of Canada
www.phac-aspc.gc.ca

Nutrition Resources

Canada's Food Guide
http://www.hc-sc.gc.ca/fn-an/food-guide-aliment/index_e.html

Canada Prenatal Nutrition Program
Community-based services that provide food, nutrition information, support, education, referral, and counselling on health issues.
www.phac-aspc.gc.ca/dca-dea/programs-mes/cpnp_main-eng.php

Dietitians of Canada
The most trusted source of information on food and nutrition for Canadians.
www.dietitians.ca

Fish Consumption
Up-to-date warnings about fish consumption across Canada on Environment Canada's website.
www.ec.gc.ca/mercury/en/fc.cfm

Nutrition Labels
Learn how to read and use nutrition labels on food.
www.healthyeatingisinstore.ca

Prenatal Nutrition
Health Canada provides prenatal guidelines on nutrition and healthy eating during pregnancy.
www.hc-sc.gc.ca/fn-an/nutrition/prenatal/index_e.html

Parenting Resources

Support programs, pregnancy outreach programs, and family resource centres offer programs and services to support families and single parents. Contact your local health office or public health nurse for more information.

Canadian Child Care Federation
Online fact sheets and resources about issues related to parenting.
1-800-858-1412
www.cccf-fcsge.ca

Dads Can
Tips and information on being a father.
1-519-685-8500 ext. 74715
www.dadscan.ca

Family Pride Canada
Information on lesbian, gay, bisexual, and transsexual family issues.
1-416-595-9230
www.uwo.ca/pridelib/family/

Father Involvement Initiative
Resources and information about father involvement.
www.cfii.ca

Multiple Births Canada
Support, education, research, and advocacy related to multiple births.
1-866-228-8824
www.multiplebirthscanada.org

Registering a Birth in Canada
How to register a birth and apply for a birth certificate.
www.servicecanada.gc.ca/en/lifeevents/baby.shtml

Pregnancy Resources

Alberta Cord Blood Banking
Public cord blood bank in Alberta.
www.acbb.ca/ACBBmain.htm

Birth Plan
A sample birth plan is available from the Society of Obstetricians and Gynaecologists of Canada.
www.sogc.org/health/pregnancy-birth-plan_e.asp

Canadian Diabetes Association
Information about diabetes.
1-800-226-8464
www.diabetes.ca

Canadian Human Rights Commission
1-888-214-1090
www.chrc-ccdp.ca

Car Safety
Transport Canada's information about being safe in a car during pregnancy.
1-888-675-6863
www.tc.gc.ca/roadsafety/safedrivers/childsafety/car/index.htm

Cord Blood Banking
The Society of Obstetricians and Gynaecologists of Canada offers information on cord blood banking.
http://www.sogc.org/health/pregnancy-cord-blood_e.asp

Due Date Calculator
www.sogc.org/health/pregnancy-calculator_e.asp

FITMOM Canada
Safe and effective approach to both pre- and post-natal fitness.
1-866-434-8666
www.fitmomcanada.com

Health Before Pregnancy
The Best Start Resource Centre's website offers information about health before pregnancy.
www.healthbeforepregnancy.ca

Healthy Pregnancy
The Public Health Agency of Canada's website provides information about healthy pregnancy.
www.healthycanadians.gc.ca/hp-gs/index_e.html

Hema-Quebec
Public cord blood bank in Québec.
www.hema-quebec.qc.ca

Lamaze International
Information about Lamaze techniques and classes (including support for breastfeeding).
1-800-368-4404
www.lamaze.org

Motherisk
*Information and guidance
for pregnant or breastfeeding
women about risks
associated with drug,
chemical, infection,
disease, and radiation
exposures.
Main Line: 1-416-813-6780
Alcohol and substance use in
pregnancy: 1-877-327-4636
Nausea and vomiting in
pregnancy: 1-800-436-8477
HIV in pregnancy: 1-888-246-5840
www.motherisk.org*

Oral Health during Pregnancy
*The Canadian Dental Association
provides oral health tips, information,
and resources to keep your family's
oral health good for life.
1-613-523-1770
www.cda-adc.ca*

Oral Health during Pregnancy
*Government of Canada
information about oral
health during pregnancy.
www.healthycanadians.gc.ca/hp-gs/
know-savoir/ora-dent_e.html*

Ovulation Calculator—Baby Center
*Online tool for figuring out when
you are likely ovulating.
www.babycenter.ca/tools/ovu/*

Pregnancy Leave and Parental Leave
*Government of Canada information
about pregnancy leave and parental
leaves.
www1.servicecanada.gc.ca/en/ei/types/
special.shtml#ParentaL2*

Pregnancy Leave and Parental Leave
*Human Resources and Skills
Development Canada's information
on length of maternity, parental,
and adoption leave in Employment
Standards legislation.
www.hrsdc.gc.ca*

Pregnancy Library
*Links to Internet pregnancy
information.
www.pregnancylibrary.com*

**Society of Obstetricians and
Gynaecologists of Canada**
*Women's health information about
pregnancy, birth control, and sexual
health.
www.sogc.org*

**Women's College Hospital, Sport
C.A.R.E.—Exercise and Pregnancy
Hotline**
*Phone line for questions about exercise
and pregnancy.
1-866-93-SPORT*

**Women's Health Matters Pregnancy
Health Centre**
*Online information about pregnancy.
www.womenshealthmatters
.ca/centres/pregnancy/index.html*

Postpartum Depression Resources

Best Start Resource Centre
*Website information on a campaign
to raise awareness about postpartum
mood disorder.
1-800-397-9567
www.beststart.org/lifewithnewbaby/
index.html*

Canadian Mental Health Association
*Information about postpartum
depression.
1-613-745-7750
www.cmha.ca/bins/content_page.
asp?cid=3-86-87-88&lang=1*

Emotional Health in Pregnancy
*www.healthycanadians.gc
.ca/hp-gs/know-savoir/
ment_e.html*

Mood Disorder Society of Canada
*Postpartum depression information.
www.mooddisorderscanada.ca*

Our Sisters' Place
*Support for women dealing with
problems related to mood and to
hormonal changes.
1-866-363-6663
www.oursistersplace.ca*

Support Groups
*Support groups for women with
postpartum depression.
1-604-255-7999
www.postpartum.org/
supportgroups.html*

Sexual Health Resources

sexualityandu.ca
*The Society of Obstetricians and
Gynaecologists of Canada's website
provides Canada's one-stop source for
information on sexual and reproductive
health, contraception, and sexually
transmitted infections.
www.sexualityandu.ca*

Canadian Federation for Sexual Health
*Information and resources on sexual
and reproductive health.*
1-613-241-4474
www.cfsh.ca

**Canadian Fertility and
Andrology Society**
*Promotes study and research about
infertility.*
1-514-524-9009
www.cfas.ca

HIV/AIDS Testing
*Public Health Agency of Canada's
information about HIV/AIDS testing.*
*www.phac-aspc.gc.ca/aids-sida/info/
4_e.html#find*

**Infertility Awareness Association of
Canada**
*Information for women having
difficulty getting pregnant or carrying
a pregnancy.*
1-800-263-2929
www.iaac.ca/en/home

**Provincial and Territorial STI/HIV/AIDS
Helpline Telephone Numbers**
*www.phac-aspc.gc.ca/std-mts/
phone_e.html*

Smoking Resources

**Canadian Cancer Society—Smokers'
Helpline**
*Free, confidential service that
provides personalized support,
advice, and information about quitting
smoking or tobacco use.*
1-877-513-5333
www.smokershelpline.ca

Go Smokefree
*Health Canada's tobacco website
provides a comprehensive range of
information and resources on
tobacco control.*
www.gosmokefree.gc.ca

Lung Association
*Information about asthma and
pregnancy, smoking and tobacco, and
smoking help phone line.*
1-888-566-5864
www.lung.ca/home-accueil_e.php

Pregnets—Smoking and Pregnancy
*Information about stopping smoking
for pregnant and postpartum women.*
1-416-535-8501 ext. 6343
www.pregnets.org

Suggested Reading

▷ *The Canadian Paediactic Society Guide to Caring for Your Child from Birth to Age Five. (2009)*
Author: Diane Sacks

> This book is the complete parenting guide from Canada's leading child and youth health care experts. Focusing on health, growth and development, safety, nutrition, and with a special section dedicated to emotional well-being, this book gives you the answers you need, from the organization that doctors and parents have relied upon for decades.

▷ *Your Child's Best Shot. (2006)*
Author: Ronald Gold. The Canadian Paediatric Society.

> This 3rd revised edition was written by Dr. Ronald Gold, a leading Canadian expert on vaccination. It answers many questions parents have about vaccination. The first version of this book was published by the Canadian Paediatric Society in 1997.

▷ *Your Baby and Child: From Birth to Age Five. 3rd edition. (2003)*
Author: Penelope Leach. Publisher: Alfred A. Knopf, New York.

> With this new, revised edition, Leach has updated her information and approach to reflect new findings in the field of child development, and to respond to the changing needs of today's families. Leach has complete respect for children and their parents; she explains development, child care, and parenting concerns clearly and with good humour.

▷ *Dr. Jack Newman's Guide to Breastfeeding. (2003)*
Authors: Jack Newman and Teresa Pitman

> This book was written by Dr. Jack Newman, a pediatrician, and Teresa Pitman, a Canadian expert on breastfeeding and International Board Certified Lactation consultant. It offers extensive practical information and encouragement on breastfeeding.

Suggested DVDs

▶ *Bringing Baby Home (2004),* The Liandrea Co.

An award-winning DVD on baby care from birth to six months. Filled with expert advice, step-by-step demonstrations, and mom-tested tips on more than 120 topics.

▶ *Dr. Jack Newman's Visual Guide to Breastfeeding* with Edith Kernerman and Jack Newman (2007)

This updated DVD explains breastfeeding, provides answers to expectant mothers, and shows health-care professionals how to recognize breastfeeding problems and help mothers solve them.

Index

A

abdomen
    after birth, 157
    discomfort during ovulation, 12
    at full term, 118
    muscles in, 95, 162–63
abuse
    during pregnancy, 67–68
    and preterm labour, 77, 83
acne, baby, 181
acupressure, 63–64
acupuncture, 63–64
aerobic exercise, 46–47, 48–49
after-pains, 161
AIDS, 11, 59–60
alcohol, health risks, 32
amniocentesis, 53, 54–55
amniotic fluid, 4, 80, 127
    in third trimester, 96
amniotic sac, 76
    rupture of, 80, 82, 96, 127, 147
anaesthetics, 139–40
analgesics, 139. *See also* pain, relief
anemia, 28, 47
antacids, 89
antibodies
    in colostrum, 109, 119
    in placenta, 119
    screening for, 51
antigens, 51
anxiety, 36. *See also* stress
Apgar score, 144, 145–46
appendicitis, 79
assisted births, 148

B

babies. *See also* embryo; fetus; newborns
    alcohol and, 32
    bathing, 176, 179–80, 196, 198
    birth registration, 168
    bleeding, 172
    bonding with, 143, 144–45
    bowel movements, 178–79
    breastfeeding, 109–13
    and breastfeeding, 107
    breasts, 169
    breathing difficulties, 172, 194
    breech, 147–48
    care of, 169–72
    clothing, 180–81
    colic, 194–95
    crying, 172, 194–97
    death of newborn, 77, 152–53
    dehydration in, 176, 178
    diarrhea, 172, 196
    in engaged position, 119
    eyes, 169, 177
    feeding, 145, 184–93 (*See also*
      breastfeeding; formula feeding)
    feeding problems, 172
    fever, 196
    first check-up, 172
    full term, 119
    hair, 169
    head, 169, 170, 183
    heart rate, 96, 122, 129, 148, 149
    immune system, 109, 119
    immunization of, 172–75
    jaundice in, 172, 175–76
    monitoring during labour, 104, 129–31
    movements of, 76, 85, 95, 96, 104, 122
    muscle tone, 145
    narcotics and, 139
    overdue, 96, 121–22
    post-term, 121–22
    premature, 30, 31, 77, 81–82, 106
    refusing food, 194
    second trimester development, 76
    seizures, 172
    sex organs, 169
    skin, 168–69, 172
    sleeping, 183–84
    smoking and, 31
    spitting up, 193–94
    temperature, 172
    tests on newborn, 144
    third trimester development, 95
    urination, 172, 178–79
    vomiting, 172, 194, 196
    weight, 95, 119
baby blues, 157–58, 159
backache
    exercise for, 50
    in late pregnancy, 119
    and preterm labour, 78
    in second trimester, 86
bacteria, 99
balance, changes in, 49
bathtub, 179
bearing down. *See* pushing
bed rest, 86, 87. *See also* rest
bereavement support, 153
bike riding, 46
birth. *See also* delivery; labour
birth canal, 127, 130, 136, 137, 140, 147, 148
birth control, 4, 13–14, 160, 163, 164–65
birth defects, 3, 32–33, 52
birthing ball, 134
birthing bars, 137
birthing rooms, 100
birth plan, 100, 101, 108, 150
births. *See also* delivery; labour
    assisted, 148
    breech, 147–48
bleeding. *See also* hemorrhage; vaginal
    discharge
    in babies, 172

hepatitis B, 51
HIV, 51
maternal serum screening, 54
on newborns, 144, 145
non-stress, 96
nuchal translucency, 54
Pap smear, 51
pregnancy, 5
purpose of, 50, 52–53
rubella, 51
syphilis, 51
of urine, 51
varicella, 51
third trimester, 36, 93–116
tiredness, 64
toenails, trimming, 180
toxemia, 150. *See also* hypertension
toxoplasmosis, 20
transcutaneous electric nerve stimulation
  (TENS), 138–39
travel
  by car, 65
  during pregnancy, 45
trimesters, 36
  first, 37–72
  second, 74–92
  third, 94–116
tubal ligation, 165
tummy time, 183
twins. *See* multiple births

U

ultrasound, 52, 53, 54, 74, 76, 80,
  82, 96, 122, 148
umbilical cord, 75, 76, 106
  blood banking, 108
underweight, and preterm labour, 80
urinary incontinence, 162
urinary tract infection, 87–88
  testing for, 51

urinating
  during first trimester, 65
  frequency, 65, 88
  problems after delivery, 162
urine
  protein in, 97 (*See also*
    hypertension)
  testing of, 51
uterus
  after delivery, 143
  and breastfeeding, 110, 151, 157,
    158–59
  contraction of, 78, 161
  and early labour, 127
  effect of massage on, 151
  during first trimester, 37
  growth of, 88
  in late pregnancy, 118
  and menstrual cycle, 12
  postpartum, 157
  role in pregnancy, 4
  in second trimester, 75
  in third trimester, 95

V

vaccines. *See* immunizations
vacuum extraction, 148
vaginal discharge, 120–21, 127,
  158–59
vaginal pain, 160–61
varicella, 51, 57
vasectomy, 165
vernix, 76
vitamins, 23–24
  importance of, 28
  vitamin D, 24–25, 185
vitamin supplements, 41
vocalization, during labour, 138
vomiting, 62–64
  in babies, 172, 194, 196

W

walking, 46, 48, 163
water
  for babies, 113
  drinking, 48, 50, 63
water breaking, 82
weaning, 112, 113
weight
  of baby, 30, 31, 32
  and body mass index, 38–40
  gain and stress, 163
  gain during pregnancy, 39–41
  of mothers, 8, 9
  and preterm labour, 80
weight control, 8–9, 29
Well Baby drop-in centres, 172
working
  physical, dangers of, 78, 84, 85–86
  during pregnancy, 30

Z

zinc, 24

Introduction

Use the space provided on page 218 to write down all the important contact information you will need **before** you go into labour. Once it's time to go to the hospital, you won't need to scramble and you can follow the action list below.

You are in labour and it's time to go the hospital when (see page 126 for more info):

- Your water breaks in a gush, or is leaking steadily.
- Your contractions are regular and five minutes apart (and the hospital is LESS than 30 minutes away).
- Your contractions are regular and 10 minutes apart (and the hospital is MORE than 30 minutes away).

NOTE: If you don't know how to measure your contractions (see page 127), or if you are still unsure, call the Labour and Delivery unit at your hospital.

What to do when you go into labour:

Action List:

- ☐ Call your ride, the ambulance or a taxi.
- ☐ Call your labour support team: partner, labour coach and/or whoever you would like with you at the hospital.
- ☐ Call your babysitter/pet sitter to arrange for care while you're in the hospital (if needed).
- ☐ Grab your suitcase (refer to page 120 for recommended items for you and your baby). Don't forget taxi or parking money.
- ☐ Celebrate! Call your family members and friends.

Contact list

Transportation

Ambulance: Phone:

Ride to hospital name: Phone: Cell:

Alternate ride to hospital name: Phone: Cell:

Taxi: Phone:

Labour support

Partner: Phone: Cell:

Labour coach name: Phone: Cell:

Support network

Babysitter name: Phone: Cell:

Pet sitter name: Phone: Cell:

Household help name: Phone: Cell:

Neighbour name: Phone: Cell:

Public health nurse name: Phone: Cell:

Breastfeeding consultant name: Phone: Cell:

Family and friends

Name: Phone: Cell:

Name: Phone: Cell:

Name: Phone: Cell:

Medical contacts

Health-care provider name: Phone: Cell:

Hospital address:

Hospital - main switchboard   Phone:

Hospital - labour and deliver unit Phone:

Pediatrician name: Phone: Cell:

List of appointments with my health-care providers

Health-care provider name	Date/Time